Community Occupational Therapy

A GUIDE TO SERVING THE COMMUNITY

Susan K. Meyers, EdD, MBA, OTR, FAOTA
RESOURCE Foundation, Inc.

JONES AND BARTLETT PUBLISHERS
Sudbury, Massachusetts
BOSTON   TORONTO   LONDON   SINGAPORE

World Headquarters

Jones and Bartlett Publishers
40 Tall Pine Drive
Sudbury, MA 01776
978-443-5000
info@jbpub.com
www.jbpub.com

Jones and Bartlett Publishers
Canada
6339 Ormindale Way
Mississauga, Ontario L5V 1J2
Canada

Jones and Bartlett Publishers
International
Barb House, Barb Mews
London W6 7PA
United Kingdom

Jones and Bartlett's books and products are available through most bookstores and online book-sellers. To contact Jones and Bartlett Publishers directly, call 800-832-0034, fax 978-443-8000, or visit our website, www.jbpub.com.

Substantial discounts on bulk quantities of Jones and Bartlett's publications are available to corporations, professional associations, and other qualified organizations. For details and specific discount information, contact the special sales department at Jones and Bartlett via the above contact information or send an email to specialsales@jbpub.com.

The author, editor, and publisher have made every effort to provide accurate information. However, they are not responsible for errors, omissions, or for any outcomes related to the use of the contents of this book and take no responsibility for the use of the products and procedures described. Treatments and side effects described in this book may not be applicable to all people; likewise, some people may require a dose or experience a side effect that is not described herein. Drugs and medical devices are discussed that may have limited availability controlled by the Food and Drug Administration (FDA) for use only in a research study or clinical trial. Research, clinical practice, and government regulations often change the accepted standard in this field. When consideration is being given to use of any drug in the clinical setting, the health care provider or reader is responsible for determining FDA status of the drug, reading the package insert, and reviewing prescribing information for the most up-to-date recommendations on dose, precautions, and contraindications, and determining the appropriate usage for the product. This is especially important in the case of drugs that are new or seldom used.

Production Credits

Publisher: David Cella
Acquisitions Editor: Kristine Jones
Associate Editor: Maro Gartside
Editorial Assistant: Teresa Reilly
Production Director: Amy Rose
Senior Production Editor: Renée Sekerak
Marketing Manager: Grace Richards
Manufacturing and Inventory Control
  Supervisor: Amy Bacus

Cover and Title Page Design: Scott Moden
Cover Image: © Blaz Kure/ShutterStock, Inc.
Composition: International Typesetting and
  Composition
Printing and Binding: Malloy, Incorporated
Cover Printing: Malloy, Incorporated

Library of Congress Cataloging-in-Publication Data
Meyers, Susan K.
  Community practice in occupational therapy : a guide to serving the community/Susan K. Meyers.
    p. cm.
  Includes index.
  ISBN 978-0-7637-6249-0 (alk. paper)
  1. Occupational therapy services. 2. Occupational therapy—Practice. 3. Community mental health services. 4. Community-based social services. I.
Title.
  RM735.M49 2010
  362.17'8—dc22
                                      2009027209
6048
Printed in the United States of America
13 12 11 10 09   10 9 8 7 6 5 4 3 2 1

Dedication

To students who encourage me to imagine possibilities for better communities and to Sam, Ethan, Lily, Lucy, and Isabel, who are the imagineers of the future.

Contents

Acknowledgments

I would like to acknowledge the following authors for their contribution to this text:

Fengyi Kuo, DHS, OTR, CPRP
Assistant Professor, Occupational Therapy
University of Indianapolis
Indianapolis, Indiana

Ann Chapleau, DHS, MS, OTR
Assistant Professor, Occupational Therapy
Western Michigan University
Kalamazoo, Michigan

Leslie Roundtree, DHSc, MBA, OTR/L
Program Director, Occupational Therapy
Chicago State University
Chicago, Illinois

Reviewers

Debra (Tiffany) Boggis, MBA, OTR/L
Assistant Professor
School of Occupational Therapy
Pacific University
Forest Grove, Oregon

Julie A. Dorsey, MS, OTR/L, CEAS
Assistant Professor
Occupational Therapy
School of Health Sciences and Human Performance
Ithaca College
Ithaca, New York

Debora Hall, MS, OTR/L
Department Chair
Occupational Therapy Assistant Program
Delaware Technical and Community College
Owens Campus
Georgetown, Delaware

Anne M. Haskins, PhD, OTR/L
Assistant Professor
Department of Occupational Therapy
School of Medicine and Health Sciences
University of North Dakota
Grand Forks, North Dakota

Beth Ann Hatkevich, PhD, OTR/L
Clinical Associate Professor
Director, Clinical and Educational Programming
    & OTD Program Admissions Chair
Department of Occupational Therapy
College of Health Science and Human Service
The University of Toledo Health Science Campus
Toledo, Ohio

Ada Boone Hoerl, MA, COTA/C
Program Coordinator and Assistant Professor
Occupational Therapy Assistant Program
Sacramento City College
Sacramento, California

Brenda Kennell, OTR/L
Clinical Assistant Professor
Department of Occupational Therapy
Winston–Salem State University
Winston–Salem, North Carolina

Kathryn M. Loukas, MS, OTR/L, FAOTA
Associate Clinical Professor
Occupational Therapy
University of New England
Portland, Maine

Jean MacLachlan, MS, OTR/L
Associate Professor
Occupational Therapy Department
Salem State College
Salem, Massachussetts

Terry Peralta-Catipon, PhD, OTR/L
Faculty
Department of Occupational Therapy
California State University–Dominguez Hills
Carson, California

Hermine Plotnick, MA, OTR/L
Associate Professor and Program Director
Department of Occupational Therapy
School of Health Professions, Behavioral and Life Sciences
New York Institute of Technology
Old Westbury, New York

Pat Precin, MS, OTR/L
Assistant Professor
Occupational Therapy
New York Institute of Technology
Old Westbury, New York

Stacy Smallfield, DrOT, OTR/L
Assistant Professor and Chair of Admissions
Department of Occupational Therapy
The University of South Dakota
Vermillion, South Dakota

Peter Talty, MS, OTR/L
Professor
Occupational Therapy
Keuka College
Keuka Park, New York

Jodi Teitelman, PhD
Associate Professor
Department of Occupational Therapy
School of Allied Health Professions
Virginia Commonwealth University
Richmond, Virginia

Barbara J. Williams, DrOT, OTR
Director
Occupational Therapy Program
University of Southern Indiana
Evansville, Indiana

Introduction

This book introduces readers to community practice and provides suggestions for developing a program to respond to community needs. It is not intended to be a comprehensive listing of all types of community practice in which occupational therapy practitioners are involved. Many exemplary programs exist in communities throughout the country where excellent occupational therapy intervention enhances quality of life for individuals and communities. Some of these programs have been published in professional publications, many are described in student papers and manuscripts, and a great many more have gone unreported.

This book evolved from thinking about the history of health care and the role of economics in our current delivery system, the resilience of occupational therapy practitioners to identify and address changing human needs over time, and my own experiences practicing in the community. I hope that sharing these ideas will encourage others to investigate opportunities that exist for occupational therapy programs in their own communities.

Chapter 1 and Chapter 2 introduce community practice and place it in historical and economic contexts. Chapter 1 is designed to frame occupational therapy in historical context with evolving health care from home environment to hospital treatment. World events, development of technology, and economic conditions have played roles in determining human needs and the resulting methods of health care delivery. Chapter 2 includes stories from practice that describe how therapists transition from working in a medical model practice to a sometimes more flexible and challenging community practice that involves working with clients in their natural environments. Meeting clients in their homes offers an opportunity to experience other cultures, which can be one of the greatest rewards of community practice. Client-centered care involving the entire family is proposed as an ideal model for community practice. Occupational therapy has many models and frames of reference for practice, accompanied by evaluation instruments and intervention strategies. These are not included here but knowledge and skill in application will carry into community practice. I believe that occupational therapy practitioners will utilize the entire spectrum of evaluation and intervention allowed by local professional regulations to provide optimal outcomes for clients.

EXPLORING THE COMMUNITY: OPPORTUNITIES FOR PRACTICE

Chapters 3 through 6 introduce community practices that have emerged over the past 30 years. Each of these chapters focuses on a particular age group and the developmental tasks associated with it. Occupational therapy practitioners may choose to remove barriers or facilitate performance around age-appropriate occupations through the community practice contexts described in these chapters, or they may consider opportunities to develop new programs in their communities. These chapters are intended to stimulate thinking and discussion about potential for community services for each age group; they do not replace in-depth study or acquired knowledge of each population.

Chapter 3 explores tasks for childhood and adolescence and gives some examples of work opportunities available in most communities with this age group. This discussion is accompanied by stories from practice as told by experienced therapists to give readers a vicarious experience of some of the benefits and challenges of community practice. Chapter 4 focuses on adulthood and Chapter 5 is devoted to aging adults. Chapter 6 discusses opportunities to provide mental health services in the community. While some of the types of community practices described in this section employ significant numbers of therapists, options for less familiar community practices are also identified.

Most of the practice options presented in Chapters 3 through 6 are well established and offered through formal organizations that may provide job security in the form of a contract, a salary, or an established method of payment for your services. Many offer benefits such as health insurance and vacations, which are important considerations for many employees. At the same time, these practice options often offer flexibility in working times and autonomy in work environment, which may be an incentive for therapists to move into community practice.

The next five chapters are designed to take a reader through the process necessary to develop a community practice. You may want to develop a practice modeled on existing ones in other areas but new to your community, or a novel practice arising from personal interests. These chapters offer suggestions and resources for program planning, financing, marketing, and evaluation.

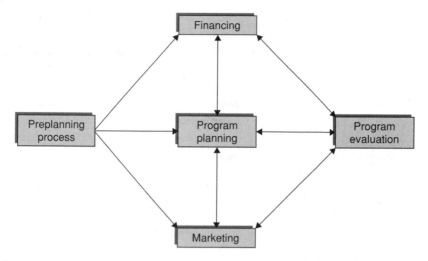

Figure FM–1 Integrating business functions provides valuable feedback to community practitioners in a changing environment.

In Chapter 7, readers can examine themselves and community opportunities as a precursor to further development of a practice. This is a process in which readers identify the motives as well as the skills and abilities to perform the actions required for successful community practice. Exploring the community for opportunities and resources completes the preliminary planning process and helps to reach a decision as to whether human needs can be addressed through an economically feasible community practice.

Having made a decision to develop a practice, you begin a second, more intensive phase of planning that involves four main functions: program development, marketing, financing, and evaluation. Although each function will be explained in detail along with resources that will assist you to move through planning and implementing your new community practice, each function will also be shown in relation to the others.

Figure FM–1 above illustrates how each function relates to and impacts the other functions of starting a community practice. The preplanning process of gathering data and reflecting on your own assets ends in a decision of whether or not you should move forward and develop your business; it also contributes data to be used in further development of your practice. Deciding on and developing your services presents a challenge when first starting your practice. This process includes making many decisions that will influence the structure and eventual success of your practice. These decisions will influence marketing plans and determine how you will finance your community practice. Integrating a fully researched program with financing, marketing, and evaluation activities provides built-in mechanisms for continuous feedback that can help you reach decisions and respond appropriately to a dynamic environment as well as to anticipated and unanticipated outcomes of your program.

The final three chapters are examples of community occupational therapy programs developed using the processes described in the earlier chapters. Each program was developed in response to a community need and was implemented and evaluated successfully.

Section

I

EXPLORING HISTORICAL AND ECONOMIC RELEVANCE OF COMMUNITY PRACTICE

Chapter 1 and Chapter 2 introduce the community practice of occupational therapy and place it in historical and economic contexts. Included are Stories from Practice that describe how therapists transition from working in an institutional practice to a more flexible, but sometimes challenging, community practice working with clients in their natural environments. One challenging experience encountered by some therapists is the transition to working in natural environments where clients' cultures differ from those familiar to the therapist. Suggestions for learning about differing cultures are demonstrated in Stories from Practice.

Whether in a hospital or in a client's home, an occupational therapy practitioner relies on professional philosophies, models, and frameworks to guide practice. Evaluation of environment and person viewed through a cultural lens facilitates intervention that enhances community participation and contributes to successful community practice.

Chapter 1

The Beginning of Community-Based Occupational Therapy

LEARNING OBJECTIVES

- Explain the foundation of occupational therapy as functional, purposeful, and meaningful to clients, and a continuing thread through the twentieth century.
- Describe the ability of occupational therapy to adapt to changes in health care.
- Explain the economic value of occupational therapy.

INTRODUCTION

Occupational therapy has it roots in the community practice of offering health-promoting occupations for persons with mental illness. Prior to the twentieth century, most health care was provided in the community, in patients' homes, and through public health services. Advances in infection control and technology gradually led to an increase in hospital services, and most medical and related health services adopted a scientific method of delivery in hospitals. As hospital based care became standard for medical treatment, healthcare costs began to increase. Over time, escalating costs created new concerns related to quality and accessibility within economic constraints. This chapter will identify some of the challenges that have emerged as health care in the United States has become more costly.

Community practice may provide an opportunity for occupational therapy practitioners to expand services to enhance quality of life, including some services not dependent upon payment by third parties. The centennial vision of the American Occupational Therapy Association suggests that occupational therapy practitioners can serve their communities by offering services of health and well-being (AOTA, 2007). As health care continues to be a significant cost in the economies of most developed countries, any services that decrease the need for hospitalization, including occupational therapy, may contribute to lowering healthcare expenditures (Timmons, 2008).

OCCUPATIONAL THERAPY ADAPTS

Prior to the twentieth century, people with mental illness were cared for in the community, and participated with caregivers and others with mental illness in work to sustain the community, exercise, and leisure activities that appeared to lessen symptoms of their illness. The idea of engaging people with disabling conditions in meaningful and purposeful occupations became a focus of the first occupational therapy practitioners (Quiroga, 1995). At the beginning of the twentieth century, as industrialization and urbanization contributed to unhealthy environments, community members with disabilities took part in activities to occupy their minds, to rehabilitate their bodies, and to give structure and meaning to their lives in the belief that participation in activities of daily living could restore them to better function and improve health (Kielhofner, 2004).

Treatment used in early occupational therapy reflected the needs of society. When farming was the main means of survival for a majority of the population, growing vegetables and fruit and raising animals for food helped sustain communities of people with mental illness. These activities occupied the minds and hands of workers and gave them a sense of satisfaction as they contributed to the survival of themselves and others. As farming became less essential to community survival, occupational therapy practitioners discovered that craft activities popular in the early twentieth century, such as needlework and woodwork, produced work that could be sold to others and enable those with disabilities to contribute to their support (Reed and Sanderson, 1999).

Although many of these occupations, such as farming, woodwork, and needlework are no longer practiced widely in much of the world, there remain communities of persons with disabilities who nonetheless must be able to sustain themselves.

A Story from Practice

On the edge of a village in Ukraine, in old buildings surrounded by farmland, sits a home for boys who are developmentally disabled. The boys range in age from toddlers to young adults and receive care and supervision from a small staff of dedicated workers. A visit to this home finds one in the midst of excited and smiling boys, eager to shake your hand and engage in a friendly conversation or ball game. Times were not always so good for this home. The building has a former life as a sanatorium and was in poor condition when the boys arrived. Over time and with support from local and international humanitarians, this home has acquired used furniture, school desks, and therapy equipment. The boys now take pride in showing visitors their rooms with tidy beds, their school and recreational areas, and their kitchen. To survive in a place where there is not enough money to buy food, clothes, or other necessities, however, these boys and their caretakers must take care of their own needs. Some of the boys farm the land or raise animals for eggs, milk, and meat. Other boys take responsibility for helping keep their home and clothes clean. Some boys learn cooking skills to assist in meal preparation. In this home, there is no occupational therapist, but the value of occupation sustains these boys in their daily living. They learn skills to help themselves and one another, and take great pride in their work.

CHANGES IN HEALTH CARE

Some of the greatest gains in the history of health care resulted from improvements in sanitation and nutrition—societal benefits that grew out of the industrial revolution. The twentieth century was well under way before modern medicine as we know it had a significant impact on the health of individuals (Folland, Goodman & Stano, 2007). Prior to the twentieth century, physicians treated most patients in their homes. Early hospitals were shunned because of their association as last resorts for people with incurable diseases or an inability to pay for care at home (Folland, Goodman & Stano, 2007). At the turn of the century, modern hospitals developed as a result of better infection control, advances in medical treatments, and urbanization, which led to a concentration of people needing and able to pay for medical care in a single location.

Treatment in psychiatric hospitals included the use of meaningful occupations under the direction of specially trained occupational therapy practitioners to help patients achieve an improved state of health (Quiroga, 1995). As soldiers returned from World War I with physical and mental disabilities, reconstruction aides were trained to restore function through rehabilitation. Although occupational therapy had long been provided in the community, physical rehabilitation resulted in occupational therapists joining other medical care providers in developing scientifically based approaches to treat people with disabilities (Folland, Goodman & Stano, 2007; Wilcock, 1998).

ECONOMICS OF HEALTH CARE

As medical treatment transitioned to hospital care, public pressure increased for more hospitals to serve both cities and rural areas. With the end of World War II, governments allocated funds for more hospital construction in areas considered to be in greatest need based on population. Government financial support of physician education followed as forecasts predicted a serious shortage of physicians. In the 1950s, advances in drugs and surgical techniques increased demand for hospital care (Dranove, 2000).

Prepaid health insurance began at the turn of the twentieth century, was offered by major industries during World War II, and served as a worker incentive as well as a cost-saving measure for the employer. Although health insurance was limited to a few employers, the mid-twentieth century booming economy, scarcity of workers, and wage restriction led to creation of worker compensation packages, including health insurance. Health insurance was a minimal cost to employers, as most people managed health costs through private payment, but healthcare benefits were an employer incentive to recruit and retain workers. In 1960, healthcare expenditures were 5.2 percent of the U.S. gross domestic product, with each individual's health care averaging $149 per year (Dranove, 2000). Through the 1960s, the majority of Americans had employer-sponsored health insurance, and those excluded by age or poverty benefited from the 1965 creation of government-funded Medicare and Medicaid (Dranove, 2000).

During the second half of the twentieth century, medical practices of all types moved into ever expanding hospital buildings. Physicians, nurses, physical and occupational therapists, and other healthcare providers saw the majority of their patients in a hospital environment. New medical professions emerged to provide technical skills needed in hospitals. An economic relationship developed between health care and the national economy. Most workers, provided health insurance by their employers, paid nothing out of pocket for their health care. As a consequence, more medical services were utilized than necessary, a practice that in some cases made people less well. The term "moral hazard" describes a situation when services or products are free or available at a very low cost and people utilize more services than they need or would choose if they had to pay for them. Consumers' un-awareness of the actual cost of health care increased demand and, although it prolonged lives, it came with a large monetary cost to society.

As healthcare costs continued to escalate in response to consumer de-mand and medical advances, managed care and legislation briefly con-tained costs in the mid-1990s (Timmons, 2008). In response to these efforts to contain costs, hospitals, pharmaceutical companies, and other health-care providers employed lobbyists to protect their economic interests. The expense of hiring and employing these lobbyists added further to health-care costs because any expense to a provider is passed on to the consumer in higher fees (Folland, Goodman & Stano, 2007). Healthcare costs again escalated as advances in medical science led to life-saving procedures that resulted in increasing numbers of individuals who required very expensive care for the rest of their lives. Gradually increasing life expectancy due to better overall health has also resulted in increasing numbers of people with high-cost needs for medicine or special care. All of these factors continue to contribute to escalating healthcare costs (Dranove, 2000).

Various countries have adopted different approaches to pay for health care. In the United States, in the mid-twentieth century, private insurance was chosen to pay for health care because it was not very expensive for the employer, provided the employer with a tax advantage, and was an incen-tive in hiring and retaining employees. Over time, this method has become very expensive for employers to maintain and contributes to production costs of all goods and services produced in the United States. In recent years employers have shifted more of the actual cost of health care to em-ployees through higher premiums, deductibles, and co-payments. Some em-ployers are unable to absorb the cost of health insurance, so it is not available to all employed residents of the United States. As a result, an estimated 47 million Americans are uninsured and another 25 million people are un-derinsured (Timmons & Cookson, 2008). Individuals without the means to pay for health care delay treatment and have poorer health as a result, which ultimately adds to the cost burden of health care in the United States. Those who have the means to pay for health care, however, may re-ceive some of the best care in the world (Timmons & Cookson, 2008). As insurance companies and government programs continue to pay for most health care in the United States, they have been able to influence where health care is dispensed, what types of services are provided, and for how long these services can be made available (Folland, Goodman & Stano, 2007). The following story illustrates the influence of the marketplace on supply and demand for occupational therapists as a result of cost structures imposed on health care.

A Story from Practice

In the early 1990s many occupational therapy practitioners worked in facilities that provided long-term care and rehabilitation to the elderly. Therapy services were compensated by private and government insurance for the elderly at a high rate. Long-term care facilities used the reimbursements for therapy to pay therapy costs, but also to pay for other things in these facilities. As an example of moral hazard, some patients who received therapy did not need the service. Demand for therapists increased as more jobs became available in long-term care facilities. Salaries for therapists rose in response to market demand, and schools of therapy expanded to provide additional therapists to supply the market. As more therapists continued to be hired, costs for care of patients in long-term care facilities became a burden on the insurance providers. As a result, toward the end of the 1990s the government placed severe restrictions on payment for rehabilitation services in these facilities. Many occupational, physical, and speech therapists left long-term care practice as a consequence of the changes in payment structure. Further consequences occurred as the job market for therapists contracted and salaries deflated in response to decreased market demand.

In countries that have chosen to have a national health service, a single government-regulated system of payment for health care provides basic care to all citizens. There are, however, limitations on the care that can be provided, and individuals must often wait to receive non-emergency care. In countries with a national health service, community practice has become an especially important cost-saving measure. Community practice may include vaccination clinics, screening for early detection of disease, and education programs publicizing the health benefits of adequate nutrition and exercise, or of avoiding substances known to cause illness. These community practices have lowered healthcare costs by avoiding or minimizing hospitalizations (Folland, Goodman & Stano, 2007).

OCCUPATIONAL THERAPY ADAPTS TO CHANGE

When most occupational therapy practitioners worked in hospitals or residential care facilities, the practice of occupational therapy developed treatment techniques that advanced the profession by responding to needs of patients and coordinating interventions with other healthcare providers. Most occupational therapy practitioners worked with other therapists in an environment that conveniently kept all necessary therapy supplies close at hand. Practicing medicine in hospitals resulted in increased professional status and recognition in the community, largely because hospitals had a reputation for providing quality medical care in a safe environment.

Mid-twentieth century practice by occupational therapy practitioners utilized treatment techniques adapted from a medical model, a reductionist approach that viewed the patient as a damaged machine that could be repaired with the proper tools (Kielhofner, 2004). Therapists specialized in treating a variety of disabling conditions with specific treatment techniques. Some therapists found this practice unsatisfying because it relied on repetitive treatments without questioning their value to clients (Wood, 2004). Occupational therapy practitioners began to have difficulty defining their profession except by describing each practitioner's work with a particular population or clinical procedure. A need arose to recapture the origins of occupational therapy and form a new practice paradigm that would define the profession for all of its practitioners (Kielhofner, 2004).

PRACTICE IN THE COMMUNITY

Wilma West declared that integration of people with disabilities back into the community could best be accomplished in the community and not in hospitals. Ann Mosey and Mary Reilly also advocated for learning living skills in the place where they were to be practiced; that is, in the community (Scaffa, 2001). In Canada, occupational therapists acknowledged the importance of taking occupational therapy out of the hospital setting in order to best address the needs of their patients. They believed that the patient's home environment, which included family, cultural values, and community resources, provided a better therapy environment than a hospital, where the focus was on illness and disability (Opzoomer & McCordic, 1973).

While occupational therapy practitioners recognized that a move to community practice would benefit patients, few programs were developed in the community through the 1970s. Occupational therapy practice continued to be associated with the type of medicine primarily provided in hospitals, and occupational therapy education programs prepared students using theories and techniques intended for practice in hospitals or clinic environments. In addition, few mechanisms existed to pay for occupational therapy provided outside the hospital or clinic.

In the 1990s occupational therapy practitioners around the world redefined themselves as professionals who prepared people with illness or disability for living life to the fullest in their own communities. Occupational therapists were returning to the foundations of their profession by listening to and addressing the needs of people who needed services. Wood (2004) describes how occupational therapists can care for clients effectively while also exercising the knowledge and techniques of modern medicine. Occupational therapy practitioners also began to see continued value in providing services perceived as important to the client, rather than prescribing treatment based on prior practice. The Canadian client-centered model for practice became instrumental in helping occupational therapy practitioners view clients as best able to determine their own futures. This led to the concept of partnership between client and practitioner to make the client's future a reality.

This convergence of economic and philosophical principles has led occupational therapy practitioners back into the community. Occupational therapy practitioners began their migration back into community practice in the 1970s by providing services in the public schools, through home healthcare agencies, and through community mental health programs. They recognized that providing their services at the natural point where skills were needed—the person's living and working environments—would make a significant contribution to bettering the lives of people with disabilities.

With this transition from institution to community, occupational therapy practitioners serve traditional roles as well as new roles in community practice. Although most practitioners provide direct care in the community, many also have become consultants to agencies, programs, and individuals. The concept of being part of a community team instead of a medical team shifts the emphasis from illness and disability to wellness and integrating differing abilities into community settings (Baum, 2007).

Occupational therapy practitioners provide needed home health interventions to persons who are undergoing fewer days of hospitalization in an effort to cut healthcare costs. Home based care has proven to be an ideal setting for occupational therapy practitioners to address the client's challenges of life in their natural context. While hospitals have adapted their facilities to accommodate persons with disabilities by providing roll-in showers and raised toilets, clients may return home only to find themselves unable to perform activities of daily living in their own environment. Meal preparation and transfers to and from one's own favorite chair become a rehabilitation challenge with significance to the client in his home. In addition to providing direct intervention, the occupational therapy practitioner becomes an educator to family members. As family members learn more about their loved one's abilities, they can help provide consistency in rehabilitation and assist in solving challenges of living at home with a disability.

Out in the community, the therapist becomes part of a team caring for a client that differs from medical teams and includes family members, friends, teachers, and employers all supporting a client's needs to fulfill valued community roles. The addition of these non-medical team members may present a challenge to a practitioner who is accustomed to working in a medical environment where there is a common language, service priorities, and payment requirements. While practicing living skills in a natural environment is an advantage, working with non-medical people to address the client's needs may be challenging. It can also be one of the greatest pleasures of working in the community.

Additional opportunities for community practice are constantly being created. Hinojosa (2007) says that many innovative opportunities exist, even in challenging economic times. Baum (2007) identifies opportunities to focus on wellness as people respond to economic necessity by learning to take greater responsibility for their own health. With continued technological advances in health care, an aging population, and rising expectations for health, there will be further demands on healthcare financing. Hospitals have continued to expand, incurring additional debt that must be recovered from patient revenues. Healthcare insurance continues to operate as a for-profit industry in the United States (Folland, Goodman & Stano, 2007). These economic conditions provide an opportunity for occupational therapy practitioners to practice in community settings where they can help promote healthier lifestyles, and perhaps ultimately help to lower healthcare costs (Timmons, 2008).

CHAPTER SUMMARY

This chapter introduces the historical significance of occupational therapy practice in the community. Changes in healthcare economics, as well as medical practices related to cost savings, provide an opportunity for community practice. With preparation for the challenges of community practice, therapists of varying levels of experience can become successful community therapists. In the following chapters, you will learn:

- Where occupational therapists currently work in the community and what they do
- How therapists prepare themselves for community practice
- How they may be paid for their services
- How to develop a community practice.

LEARNING ACTIVITIES

Learning activities are provided to guide your application of the contents of this chapter, which focused on the history of occupational therapy, including healthcare and economic factors that influence occupational therapy practice.

Write answers to these questions in a journal and save them for discussion with others or to document your thought processes as you develop a community practice.

1. Relate the history of occupational therapy as a service adaptive to individual and community needs throughout the twentieth century.
2. Identify current healthcare economic conditions and give examples of why health care in the United States has become so costly. How can community practice help contain these costs?
3. In the Occupational Therapy Centennial Vision, one role of occupational therapy practitioners is to offer services of health and well-being. How would offering these services benefit you, the profession, and your community?
4. Relate cost savings that can be achieved through preventive services—a practice used in single-payer healthcare systems—to occupational therapy services that can be offered in community practice.
5. In this chapter the term "moral hazard," taken from economics, describes disincentives that occur when insurance payments increase use of unnecessary services. Explain how moral hazard relates to your professional code of ethics and how you would guard against this in practice.
6. Explain why the promotion and maintenance of health and wellness through engagement in community, as either a service provider or a volunteer, makes economic sense.

REFERENCES

American Occupational Therapy Association (2007). AOTA Centennial vision and executive summary. *The American Journal of Occupational Therapy, 61* (6) 613–614.

Baum, C. (2007). Achieving our potential (farewell presidential address). *The American Journal of Occupational Therapy, 61* (6) 615–623.

Dranove, D. (2000). *The economic evolution of American health care: From Marcus Welby to managed care.* Princeton: Princeton University Press.

Folland, S., Goodman, A.C., & Stano, M. (2007). *The economics of health and health care (5th ed.).* Upper Saddle River, NJ: Prentice Hall.

Hinojosa, J. (2007). Becoming innovators in an era of hyperchange. (Eleanor Clarke Slagle Lecture). *The American Journal of Occupational Therapy, 61* (6) 629–639.

Kielhofner, G. (2004). *Conceptual foundations of occupational therapy (3rd ed.).* Philadelphia, PA: F.A. Davis.

Opzoomer, A. & McCordic, L. (1973). Occupational therapy: A change of focus. *Canadian Journal of Occupational Therapy, 40,* 125–129.

Quiroga, V.A.M. (1995). *Occupational therapy: The first 30 years 1900–1930.* Bethesda, MD: American Occupational Therapy Association.

Reed, K.L. & Sanderson, S.N. (1999). *Concepts of occupational therapy (4th ed.).* Baltimore, MD: Williams & Wilkins.

Scaffa, M. (2001). *Occupational therapy in community-based practice settings.* Philadelphia, PA: F.A. Davis.

Timmons, N. Growing ranks of the elderly add to age-old costs dilemma. *The Financial Times,* July 2, 2008.

Timmons, N. & Cookson, C. Sense of crisis prevails as money fails to revive an ailing system. *The Financial Times,* July 1, 2008.

Wilcock, A.A. (1998). *An occupational perspective of health.* Thorofare, NJ: Slack Inc.

Wood, W. (2004). The health, mind and soul of professionalism in occupational therapy. *The American Journal of Occupational Therapy, 58* (3) 249–257.

Chapter 2

Principles to Guide Community Practice

LEARNING OBJECTIVES

- Relate principles of temporal adaptation, challenge and support, and personal safety to community practice.
- Explain relevance of cultural awareness and sensitivity for home based services.
- Show how environmental factors contribute to client centered care.

INTRODUCTION

This chapter will describe how the practice of occupational therapy in the community may differ from occupational therapy practice in a hospital setting. In community practice, occupational therapy practitioners are often guests in the homes of clients, and need to remain sensitive to the different lifestyles and cultures they may encounter. You will learn how occupational therapy practitioners keep themselves safe as they provide services in the community. You will enhance your understanding of client centered care and community based practice as natural extensions of the philosophic base of occupational therapy.

An occupational therapy practitioner who moves from hospital based practice to community based practice may encounter many challenges, as well as develop a renewed appreciation of the value occupational therapy has to enhance quality of life through community participation. Among the challenges for an occupational therapy practitioner transitioning to community practice are working autonomously, defining standards of care and productivity, and finding support from other service providers.

HOW IS COMMUNITY PRACTICE DIFFERENT?

Defining community practice can be a challenge. We could define community practice by considering practice location, sources of payment for services delivered, elements of professional autonomy, or social justice. If we use location to define community practice of health care, then we could include any service delivered outside the hospital or medical clinic environment. We could also define community practice as any service delivered that does not utilize payment sources established for health care. Hospital or clinic based practice generally includes services that are paid for by money allocated for health care by some type of private or government sponsored healthcare insurance. Community practice is generally paid for through other sources, which may include local, state, or federal funds unrelated to health care; nonprofit funds, or private payment by clients. The problem with using payment as a means of defining community practice is that some service delivery occurring outside medical institutions may be paid for by health insurance, particularly home health and some services for children and aging adults.

Another possibility for defining community practice might include professional autonomy and control of the work situation. In most medical treatment environments, occupational therapy practitioners treat patients upon physician referral and are accountable to the employing organization's standards of care and productivity (Hinojosa, 2007). In community practice clients are often seen in their homes, may be referred for services by non-medical persons, and the standards of care and productivity may be determined by the service provider. One problem with this definition of community practice, however, is that some community organizations such as schools and home care services set standards of care and productivity for services. Occupational therapy practitioners working in these settings may have little input into how these standards are established. Social justice as a method of defining community practice arises from the notion of identifying and solving problems of people who are disadvantaged by existing social, political, or economic constraints. This includes contexts such as schools or other educational institutions, neighborhood associations, and agencies that work and provide services on behalf of residents organized by location or by common interest, such as cultural, social, political, health, or economic issues (Strand, Marullo, Cutforth, Stoecker & Donohue, 2003).

Any definition of community practice comes with exceptions. Most often the institutions I identify as community based practices in the following chapters are schools, workplaces, or community organizations that serve specific populations. Payment for these services comes from local or federal government budgets not allocated to provide health care, or are paid for by clients or others in the community. Most, but not all, community practices described arise from a sense of social justice and a need to provide services to underserved people. Community practice encompasses a wide variety of practice options, usually arising from the needs of individuals or groups of people living in the same area who share public services and have a common interest. The intention of such services is to enhance quality of life for those in the community. This intention resonates with the centennial vision of the American Occupational Therapy Association (2007) to provide services for health and well-being through occupational therapy services.

COMMUNITY PRACTICE CONSIDERATIONS

Certain skills and attitudes greatly contribute to success in community practice: time management, creativity, autonomy, cultural awareness, and personal safety. Each of these will be described and examples given of their application in community practice.

Temporal Adaptation

To begin looking at differences between hospital based and community based practice, we will consider temporal adaptation. Kielhofner (1997) described temporal adaptation as the process of adjusting to temporal changes in living skills or to changes made over the life span. Our focus will be on temporal adaptation to work when moving from a highly structured environment to one that may have few externally provided structures. Typically an occupational therapy practitioner in a hospital environment begins every day at the same time. Some institutions use time clocks to regulate arrival and departure times for workers. Using Kielhofner's (2002) model of human occupation, a typical workday begins with some sort of habitual performance that requires little concentration. Arising and preparing for work, an occupational therapy practitioner may not need to choose her work clothing, as a uniform is worn. Breakfast is followed by transportation to work by car or public transportation; even the route does not vary unless traffic or road construction interferes. Once the occupational therapy practitioner arrives at her place of work she begins her work routine. There may be variability in the order in which the occupational therapy practitioner performs her work, and new clients may present challenges, but the rhythm of the workday usually remains constant. Temporal adaptation may not be a significant challenge to the hospital based occupational therapy practitioner, as she arrives at work at the same time each day, takes lunch or breaks at regular intervals, and leaves work each day about the same time. Often, support staff schedules clients, and therapy practitioners must merely monitor the schedule and limit their time with each client to assure that they see all scheduled clients. For a hospital based occupational therapy practitioner, time may be managed for her rather than by her.

In contrast, for the occupational therapy practitioner working in community practice, there may be little routine to most days. She is frequently autonomous in scheduling her clients. She will usually know how many clients will need to be seen each week as set by an employer or her own need for revenue production, but even this is subject to an occasional change of plans. Although our hospital based and community based occupational therapy practitioners may awaken at the same time each workday, their routines differ significantly once they have completed self care in the morning. The community based service provider may go to a different location each day to perform her work. The time she schedules to see her clients and the length of each session may vary. Her work times may vary, breaks for lunch or other purposes may be at a different time each day, and some days she may have to eat as she travels from one home to the next. Temporal adaptation is a challenge for the occupational therapy practitioner working in the community. She will need to become skilled at scheduling and managing her time each day and throughout a week of work.

A Story from Practice

Fran, an occupational therapy practitioner in community practice, works for a government-supported early intervention program. She receives referrals from a regional agency for children who have been evaluated for developmental delays and who have been identified as needing occupational therapy. Each week Fran may see 15 to 25 children who need her services. Most children will be seen one time a week but some will be seen twice a week. Before the first visit to a child, Fran must contact the parents by phone to arrange a mutually agreeable time to visit their home for therapy. One scheduling challenge she has is accommodating the needs of children in this age group to take naps. She knows that most children nap at about the same time each afternoon and none of the mothers want to schedule therapy during nap time. Most parents prefer a morning session when their

*children are most attentive to therapy, but with many children needing her serv-
ices, Fran knows that she will need to see some children in the afternoon. Another
challenge is that some of the children Fran treats attend preschool programs every
day because parents work outside the home. She then must schedule services for these
children at a time convenient for their preschools.*

*In this developmental program each therapy session lasts one hour, but it may
take Fran up to another hour to travel to the next child's home or preschool. Fran
attempts to organize her visits so that she can provide services to children living in
a particular area of the city on the same day to minimize travel time between
homes. When a child becomes three years of age, he is no longer eligible to receive
this community service and a new client is added to Fran's schedule. Fitting a new
child into her existing schedule can be difficult as the new child's therapy session
needs to be scheduled to be agreeable with parents. Scheduling therapy visits in the
community can be complicated.*

*Occupational therapy practitioners who provide community care to children
enrolled in this program are paid for each individual visit. If a visit does not occur,
Fran does not get paid. Therefore an additional challenge is establishing a schedule that is financially feasible when there are cancellations due to a child's illness,
a family vacation, or when a mother forgets her child's occupational therapy appointment and simply is not at home when the service provider arrives. These are
typical temporal challenges for an occupational therapy practitioner providing
services in the community.*

This story illustrates some of the challenges in organizing for community practice. Although not all community practice requires self-
scheduling, organizing, and logically planning visits to economize on
time and travel expenses, these skills may be important to success for
many in community practice. Consider your own organizational skills.
This will help determine where you may find the greatest success in community practice.

Clinical Challenge and Support

In the past, most occupational therapy practitioners began their careers in
hospital settings because this is where the majority of jobs could be found.
In hospitals, there were usually many occupational therapy practitioners,
some with years of experience, to serve as role models and help a new therapist improve her skills (Wilcock, 1998). When an occupational therapy
practitioner, even one with many years of experience, discovered a client

problem that was challenging to her, she could receive assistance in finding solutions to the problem in a supportive work environment.

There have been some changes in this scenario. As a result of shorter hospital stays and a changed structure of reimbursement for therapy services, fewer occupational therapy practitioners work in hospital settings, and the pace of work means there are fewer opportunities to discuss clients with others. In a hospital environment, however, there are usually other therapists, nurses, or physicians available, and most hospitals have a library or other reference sources available on site to help an occupational therapy practitioner find information to solve a client problem. In addition, efforts to improve service efficiency mean that most occupational therapy practiced in hospitals follows treatment protocols focused on specific treatment techniques (Hinojosa, 2007).

By comparison, an occupational therapy practitioner working in the community will most often work independently. This does not mean, however, that a community based therapist lacks resources to help solve problems that arise in practice; solutions may just be less easily available than in a hospital. A community based service provider must build her own professional supports by identifying community resources that provide additional knowledge or experience to help her with solving client problems. Occupational therapy practitioners in the community are often in contact with colleagues who practice with the same age or diagnostic group. They may communicate by phone or e-mail, or periodically meet face to face to learn and share. Some community therapists work for agencies that hold regularly scheduled meetings that bring all occupational therapy practitioners together in a single place to be informed of new procedures, provide continuing education, and to network with each other. The use of the internet expands a community of therapists to include those who may live far away but have similar clinical concerns. The internet also provides options for continuing to learn about research and clinical treatment. A community based occupational therapy practitioner may have to use different strategies than a colleague who is hospital based to find resources when challenges arise, but the resources are equally available.

Supplies and Equipment

A hospital setting may conveniently offer the latest therapy supplies and equipment. This equipment normally remains within the hospital because it may be expensive and not portable. Occupational therapy practitioners working in a hospital can quickly and easily access equipment and supplies needed for treatment, and many plan client interventions around these resources. Activities of daily living, such as using a toilet or a bathtub, may be practiced in adapted bathroom facilities in the hospital. If kitchen facilities are available in the hospital, clients can practice instrumental activities of daily living such as meal preparation. Such a kitchen may have many adaptations that accommodate clients' performance challenges. The occupational therapy practitioner identifies the client's needs and then teaches the client how to meet these needs through intervention in the hospital's accommodating environment.

By contrast, in a community setting, the equipment available for use with clients is what is found in their own homes or what the occupational therapy practitioner brings with her to the client's home. This can be both a challenge and benefit of community practice. Working with a client in her own home on living skills that are important to her demonstrates the full potential of occupational therapy. In community settings, living skills are learned and practiced in the place where they must be performed and the occupational therapy practitioner does not need to wonder whether interventions provided in an adapted environment will readily transfer to the client's home environment. Most occupational therapy practitioners who work in the community enjoy problem solving with clients about how to make their homes safer and more accessible. Together they work on making therapy a daily part of the clients' lives as they become more independent and capable of performing personally meaningful activities.

In the hospital setting, a client is often treated in isolation from family or other people who may be in a position to help them when they return home. In community practice, family members and supportive caregivers become part of the therapy process. Establishing goals and intervention are collaborative efforts among all of the people who will share community living with the client. The occupational therapy practitioner observes the environmental barriers that exist in the client's home; she sees and hears the impact a client's condition may have on family members and can address these concerns through her intervention. The absence of elaborate therapy equipment and an adapted environment may appear to be a disadvantage until one considers that most people who receive occupational therapy do not have extensive adaptations made to their home to accommodate disability, nor do the majority of clients use specialized equipment in their homes. The reason for this may be economic, as the family or the client may not be able to afford home modifications or special equipment. Many people with disabilities, however, dislike the way special equipment looks, or their family members may object to changing the home to accommodate a person with a disability.

A Story from Practice

Fran, who works with young children in their homes, transports her therapy equipment with her. Because of the age of her clients, her car contains bags of developmental toys and sanitizing wipes to clean the toys between uses by different children. She makes some of her own therapy equipment with supplies she purchases at fabric or hardware stores. Fran is always looking for toys that will meet the needs of her clients at resale shops and yard sales and happily accepts donations from friends whose children have outgrown their toys. She looks for inexpensive items that develop skills and are easily cleaned between uses.

This story illustrates how many community service providers search for therapy supplies and ideas continuously in the community, but allow flexibility and creativity into their search.

Of all the differences between hospital based and community based occupational therapy practitioners, the biggest difference may be autonomy in practice. The community based therapy practitioner is responsible for planning her schedule, her work hours, and client intervention, as well as fulfilling the documentation and billing requirements for her services. She does not have to work the same hours every day and can adjust her schedule to accommodate her personal needs. Like her hospital based colleague, however, she remains responsible for her clients' quality of care and must provide intervention demonstrated to provide optimal outcomes. Whether an occupational therapy practitioner works in an institution or in the community, many aspects of service delivery are the same. A professional code of ethics applies to all practitioners, who must also remain current on healthcare trends and mindful of the latest research about the efficacy of interventions. The choice to practice in the community is based on an occupational therapy practitioner's knowledge of herself and her abilities, as well as her preference for routine or variety.

Personal Safety

Service providers often must go into communities or neighborhoods with which they are unfamiliar. An occupational therapy practitioner working in the community and visiting client homes must know how to address environmental safety issues and take responsibility for her own personal safety. Personal safety may be a special concern to therapists working in neighborhoods where she needs to be wary of strangers or criminal activity. Sometimes an occupational therapy practitioner knows she will be visiting a client in a neighborhood that is considered unsafe. What is an unsafe neighborhood? It may be an area where illicit drug sales are known to occur and where there is significant drug use by area residents. Crime rates, including violent crimes, may be higher in certain areas of the city. Most of these concerns are centered in areas where residents experience low levels of income and education along with high rates of unemployment. Since clients needing home based occupational therapy come from a cross-section of society, they may live in neighborhoods at risk for crime. Although some providers choose not to deliver services in areas where they feel unsafe, the majority of home care therapists go where a need exists, exercising caution to protect themselves in the process.

A Story from Practice

As I made my visits into a particular neighborhood where people were very poor, where cars stood abandoned, and few people seemed to be out and about, I became anxious. I knew from reading the newspaper that crimes occurred frequently in this neighborhood and I worried that I might become a victim of one. Friends and acquaintances advised me to be careful if I visited clients in this neighborhood. I was thoroughly frightened about going to this neighborhood to see clients, but I learned some interesting things as I continued to visit there.

A sticker on my car's windshield indicated I was working for a home healthcare agency, but I did not realize at first how meaningful this was to my personal safety. As I made my first visits, I saw people watching me from their windows and sometimes from the street, which made me uneasy, but no one bothered me. As I got to know my client, she told me it was difficult to get a therapist to come to her home because of her bad neighborhood and I admitted I had been concerned about this. She asked me: "Have you seen people watching you as you come to my house? They know from the sticker on your car windshield that you are coming here to help me and they are watching to protect you."

Just as a sticker posted on the car windshield identified me as someone who provided care, sometimes uniforms or other identifiable symbols worn or carried to homes also provide this type of protection for community therapists. Since community practice therapists work according to scheduled visits mutually arranged with clients, the therapist is expected to arrive at a specific time. The client, and sometimes the client's neighbors, will often watch for her arrival and departure. Letting your client know when to expect you helps in assuring personal safety. Letting a colleague know where you are going, and what time you are scheduled to arrive and depart is another good personal safety practice.

A Story from Practice

In one particular community mental health practice in a large city, the office shared by all service providers utilized a schedule board where each person wrote his or her schedule for the day. We wrote the phone numbers of clients to be visited next to the time we were scheduled to be in each client's home. When a service provider had concerns about the safety of a visit, he or she would indicate this concern on the schedule board and would alert all of the others in the office of this concern. The arrangement was that after a visit of concern the service provider would phone the office to say he or she had left the client's home safely. If she or he did not phone the office to say the visit was completed safely, a colleague from the office would phone the service provider or the client's home to make certain that the visit was safely concluded. If no one answered, a predetermined procedure sent either police or others to the client's home to be certain the service provider was safe.

Cell phones are a valuable safety tool for healthcare providers practicing in the community as they can be pre-programmed to call for emergency help. Phones allow community service providers to phone clients to tell them to expect a late arrival or to ask the client to watch for them out the window. They provide convenience, but more importantly cell phones provide safety for the community health care providers who carry them.

When out walking in the community, it is important to always remain alert to your surroundings, even in neighborhoods considered safe. It is important to follow your instincts; if you feel unsafe, be extra alert or seek safety in a public place. Crowded or more public places generally feel safer than isolated spots.

A Story from Practice

While in community practice, I visited one client who lived in an area isolated by many superhighways that had cut his neighborhood off from most of the rest of the community. To reach his home, I had to travel under a tangle of highways through underground walkways. There were rarely any other people around when I had to walk through these underground walkways, so I would look around both sides of the walkway before going underground then I would walk through very quickly with my cell phone in hand. This was stressful, although the idea of walking through tunnels may have been more frightening than the actual walk. I eventually found a less direct above-ground route to my client's home that felt safer to me, even though there still were very few other people along this route. Just remaining constantly aware of one's environment is important to assure safe work conditions.

When working with mental health clients in community practice, service providers must exercise some additional safeguards. When entering a client's home for the first time, it is important to maintain direct access to the door. If a client is agitated, do not let the client stand between you and the door. If you feel unsafe, leave the home. You can always return later when the client has calmed down.

If the client is unstable, or if there is another concern for personal safety, do not visit the client's home alone. Most community mental health practices allow for service providers to pair with a colleague to visit a client when there may be a concern for personal safety.

A Story from Practice

After many months of uneventful visits to a woman in the community, my client's husband suddenly posed a threat to her safety as well as my own. During a visit, my client showed me bruises on her neck and told me that her husband had attempted to kill her. I asked the client if her husband was in the home with us and she answered in the affirmative. I considered the risk of harm to my client and myself ongoing, and I asked the client to leave her home with me. Once we were out of the home, I phoned the police on behalf of the client. Although in time this threat lessened, the client continued to live with her husband and I still needed to visit her. I asked a male colleague to accompany me for a few visits. My male colleague was able to talk to my client's husband about the behavior that threatened my client's safety. After a few accompanied visits, the problem seemed to resolve and I returned to visiting my client alone.

Personal safety is one aspect of community practice that must be managed. There are many strategies to make the community a very safe environment in which to work. Having confidence in oneself, knowing how to calm agitated clients, knowing how to get help when needed, and remaining alert while traveling to and from clients' homes—as well as while in their homes—will contribute to safe practice in the community.

CULTURAL AWARENESS: THE THERAPIST IS A GUEST IN A CLIENT'S HOME

One of the best features of community practice is the opportunity to visit clients in their own homes and communities. This also provides an occupational therapy practitioner with a challenge to become comfortable in cultural environments that differ from her own. It has been found that one of the greatest barriers to effective care in a multicultural environment is value conflict between therapist and client (Fitzgerald, Mullavey-O'Byrne & Clemson, 1997).

Culture is defined as the attitudes, ideas, beliefs, and customs that are shared by a group of people (Fatehi, 2008; Fitzgerald, et al., 1997). A common misperception is that culture defines a group of people who are of the same race or ethnicity (Litterst, 1985, Bourke-Taylor & Hudson, 2005). People who share race or ethnicity may belong to different cultural groups and may consider being classified by their ethnicity or race as being stereotyped. If we are to establish a therapeutic relationship with our clients, it is important to observe and learn from them and not label them by racial or other characteristics.

Culture is often studied through ethnography (Bourke-Taylor & Hudson, 2005). Ethnography is research designed and implemented to improve understanding of people bounded into a group by common characteristics (Hesse-Biber & Leavey, 2006). An ethnographer seeks to understand a group by examining relationships among members of the group; their use of technology; their behaviors, such as rituals and social practices; and their economic, political, and religious characteristics (Creswell, 2007). Phenomenologists also study people, but focus on understanding the lived experiences of a person or a specific group of people (Hesse-Biber & Leavey, 2006). In order to appreciate activities from the client's perspective, it is valuable for an occupational therapy practitioner to learn from the client what it is like to live in a specific place and time while dealing with a disruption in functional performance. Both ethnography and phenomenology, research approaches used by occupational therapy practitioners and other social scientists, provide a means to learn about cultural groups (Crabtree & Miller, 1998). Practicing occupational therapy in the community using knowledge and techniques from these research approaches is valuable to understanding a client's culture. By observing and listening to stories told by clients and their families of their experiences, we can provide intervention that is meaningful in the client's cultural context.

A different approach to understanding culture is described by Bonder, Martin, and Miracle (2004). They describe culture as being responsive to change in the environment while at the same time providing an individual with structure for understanding how to adapt to those changes. They maintain that culture is learned from family and the institutions that bind a community together and give it identity. It is based on local beliefs, values, and rules designed to maintain order. Culture includes rituals and habits that give meaning to the individual within the group.

As one moves from one cultural group to another, however, a different set of values, rules, and meanings may need to be understood in order to adapt and function within a new environment. Cultural adaptation applies to clients as well as service providers, and requires modifications in cognition, habits, and roles as they differ from those inherited from family and community of origin. In transition from one culture to another, a person will use values of their culture of origin to make sense of a new culture. The process of cultural adaptation results in a person changing some of his or her behaviors to fit into a new cultural environment (Bonder, Martin & Miracle, 2004).

A Story from Practice

When I began working as an occupational therapist in an area of a major city with a large immigrant population, I found that each day required transition from one culture to another to work effectively with my clients. My own culture includes beliefs about fairness for all people regardless of gender, race, or ethnicity. The rights of each person to choose what he wants independently is not only reflective of my country of origin, but of Western-influenced occupational therapy. Enculturation to Judeo-Christian religious traditions helps form the cultural lens through which I view the world.

In my practice in the city, I encountered Hindu women from India, Muslim men and women from Bangladesh, Jewish women from Eastern Europe, and men and women from Vietnam, Hong Kong, Ireland, and Somalia. Each person lived in a culture different from my own with different beliefs about roles of men and women in society, religion, functional performance, and independence. These cultural differences often challenged my own beliefs, but to function effectively as an occupational therapist in this community I had to learn about the culture of each of my clients.

Learning to listen without the interference of personal bias is difficult. Failing to understand the culture of others, however, can prove an obstacle to effective community practice (Royeen & Crabtree, 2006).

Cross-cultural practice in occupational therapy should reflect standards of social justice in which all people who need service receive it in a culturally sensitive manner. Awareness of one's own culture and biases toward others' cultures is the first step in developing cultural competency (Bourke-Taylor & Hudson, 2005). Although cultural competence is desirable for all occupational therapy practitioners no matter where they work, it has special meaning when practice is conducted in the homes of clients. After one becomes aware of one's own culture, the next step to acquiring cultural competency is to learn about other cultures. Using the methods of ethnography and phenomenology, the occupational therapist observes and questions, reads, and then asks more questions.

A Story from Practice

In my community practice I wanted to learn as much as possible about the culture of my clients. The richness of this learning experience contributed to the pleasure I found in my work and became a mutually beneficial exchange of ideas that led to better therapeutic relationships with my clients. They learned how to adapt their lifestyle to their disabilities through occupational therapy, and I learned about how people live differently depending on cultural beliefs, values, and customs. I began learning about my clients' cultures by observing customs in the homes I visited. Sometimes a client informed me of the behaviors expected by her culture and sometimes I had to observe or ask what I should do. Many of my clients took their shoes off in their homes. They sometimes told me that I didn't need to take my shoes off, but to establish a respectful relationship, I took my shoes off when I entered their homes. Sharing food or beverage may have been valued social behavior in my client's culture, and for me to refuse this offering would be culturally insensitive. The clothing I wore to some of my client's homes was specifically chosen to respect their tradition of modesty. When I made these accommodations to their culture, my clients often stated their appreciation of my actions. They would never have asked me to dress a certain way or to engage in some of the customs of their culture because such a direct request would have been uncomfortable for them. If my intervention suggestions were to be agreeable to my clients, however, they had to trust that I was sensitive to what they could and could not do within their cultural context. I discovered early in this experience that clients might not tell me that my intervention suggestions could not be implemented, because they did not want to offend me; they just didn't act on them. Once a good relationship was established with a client, she would tell me more about her culture and what interventions could be done and which could not.

One client, a mother of two very young children, had come to this large city as a child and had been educated in its public schools. Prior to her arranged marriage she had been employed in a job she loved. With marriage she was required to give up her job along with her contacts with friends from work and school. As a result, she became very depressed and in a suicide attempt suffered permanent physical injuries. Together we talked about her finding some activities outside her home that were meaningful and pleasurable to decrease her depression. I knew of a

> *group of mothers that met weekly to engage in socialization and developmental play with their young children and suggested this as an option for my client. She told me this would not work for her as she could socialize only with women of her religion and within her neighborhood. This information helped me discover a more suitable mother-child group for this client, which she found helpful in coping with her depression. She would participate in this local group with the full approval of her community and her family without any feelings of anxiety. This experience helped me to become more culturally sensitive, but also gave me insight into how this young mother struggled to adapt from the culture of her youth to her family's culture of origin and their expectations of behavior for her roles as wife, mother, daughter, and family member.*

This example shows how occupations are interpreted through a lens of culture. The roles of a person may change with age or marital status. Within a given culture, gender roles may be rigidly defined and restrict occupational choice. In the example above, the woman was able go to school and work outside the home until marriage, but once married, these activities are forbidden within her culture.

Disability may complicate performance of gender roles expected by one's culture and result in dissatisfaction with life. When a woman whose culturally expected role includes care of home and family acquires a disability, she may no longer be able to perform expected tasks or roles. As a result she may feel that she is letting her family down by not meeting cultural expectations for her gender. This can lead to feelings of worthlessness within her family and her community. Her husband may experience dissatisfaction with his wife if he must now assume some of the tasks or roles she previously performed and which he considers inappropriate for a man.

By the same token, when a man loses his ability to work outside the home due to illness, injury, or job loss due to economic conditions, his cultural role as provider for his family is compromised. His wife may need to work outside the home to support their family, which may influence how each perceives the other as well as how they see themselves. Within the partner relationship as well as within the cultural community, the man may feel he is worthless if he cannot provide an income for his family. His wife may feel resentment if she must do all the work inside the home and provide an income from work outside the home. Conversely, she may feel empowered by her ability to provide all that is needed for her family. This may be a culturally new and possibly dangerous situation for a woman in a male-dominated culture.

Gender role shifts will have different meanings in different cultures. Regardless of which culture is involved, an occupational therapy practitioner working in community practice will encounter role shifts that may create conflicts within a marital relationship. The occupational therapy practitioner working in a multicultural practice needs to learn about differing roles, habits, and rituals for men and women from one culture to another in order to be effective working with families adapting to illness or injury of a loved one. This is accomplished through client centered interactions. The occupational therapy practitioner must listen to the client and learn about the client's needs and desires, and then develop intervention through a process of negotiated understanding.

COMMUNITY PRACTICE IS CLIENT CENTERED PRACTICE

As a practitioner begins to provide occupational therapy in the community, a medical model of practice, which is often used in institutions, does not seem appropriate. A medical model of practice is focused on finding the medical, physical, or psychological problem and "fixing" it. This approach to therapy is reinforced by reimbursement policies that strive to minimize cost of care by shortening treatment times (Folland, Goodman & Stano, 2007). Healthcare providers treat a client with medicine, surgery, manipulation, or other applications of technical expertise. Within the medical model of specialized care, occupational therapy practitioners may provide many different interventions, including adaptive equipment, safe and comfortable seating and splinting, as well as interventions that strengthen muscles and increase endurance—all while focusing on occupations valued by the client. These interventions, applied in various hospital and institutional settings, prepare clients to become more independent, usually with the objective of returning to their homes. Recognizing that occupational therapy practitioners following a medical model in a hospital incorporate client centered components into treatment, reimbursement practices require intervention protocols based on evidence that may be less favorable toward allocating time to understanding client needs. A challenge for the occupational therapy practitioner is finding time to incorporate educating the client to his functional abilities, listening to his needs and desires, and developing evidence-based intervention protocols within the constraints of a hospital's productivity and reimbursement schedules (Baum, 1998; Tickle-Degnan, 2002).

The *International Classification of Functioning, Disability and Health* (ICF) describes the main focus of medical model treatment as identifying and curing a disability (World Health Organization, 2001). Kielhofner (2004) states that the medical model, concentrated on diagnosis and treatment of disability, may be at odds with occupational therapy's concern for a person with a disability living a meaningful life. Occupational therapy practitioners identify client centered care, in which the client selects treatment with personal meaning, as an important component of the occupational therapy paradigm (Kielhofner, 2004). Within a hospital setting, an occupational therapy practitioner may be challenged to find time to identify what the client's home needs might be, and a visit to a client's home for observation is often impractical and not financially justified. Furthermore, a client with a recently acquired disabling condition may not have any idea what challenges await him once he leaves the hospital. Even if an occupational therapy practitioner were to discuss environmental constraints to functional performance with him, the client may not be able to identify community living challenges.

Further constraints to effective client centered practice in hospitals or other institutions are time and economics. Institutions incur high costs for inpatient care, just knowing what a client's home needs will be; it includes acknowledging that the client has the right to make informed decisions about his care. Limited contact time in a hospital environment, however, may prevent a service provider and client from reaching a mutual understanding or a fully informed decision about what the client's future needs may be in a home environment.

For many occupational therapy practitioners inspired by the potential for client centered care, the lack of time and resources to establish relationships with clients within an institutional environment provides the catalyst for transitioning to community practice. When we shift occupational therapy services from the hospital to the community, client centered care becomes a natural basis on which to build treatment. The occupational therapy practitioner observes the client within his natural environment and usually has more time to develop an understanding of the client's performance needs and constraints. Objects and any architectural barriers in the client's home, along with the people who add richness, joy, or stress within that environment are all tangible. By visiting and spending time in a client's home and community, the occupational therapy practitioner can consider intervention options from within an economic and cultural understanding of the client's circumstances.

Client centered occupational therapy is a collaborative process between client and occupational therapy practitioner. The client and his family are respected and share equally in decisions (Sumsion, 1999; Law & Mills, 1998). This is a paradigm shift from a medical model practice, in which an occupational therapy practitioner is the expert and determines what intervention is best for a client. Client centered care requires that an occupational therapy practitioner observe and listen to the client's wants and needs, and only then offer intervention alternatives from among which a client may choose whatever is relevant to his life. In community practice all of this observation and discussion happens within the context of the client's own environment.

A Story from Practice

When working in the community, I discovered that intervention was made relevant by events that occurred in my clients' lives. A client who normally functioned at a high level of independence rather suddenly experienced stress related to her child's poor performance in school. This led the client to a brief period of hospitalization to assess medication for her depression. My community job stressed continuity of care so that when a client went into the hospital, we continued to work collaboratively while planning for discharge to her home. In order to assess situations that might interfere with a successful discharge, the client and I planned to spend an afternoon in her home. During this visit, I observed that her formerly organized and tidy living room was messy and full of unopened mail, her kitchen was full of dirty dishes, and dirty clothes covered the floor of her bedroom. My client sighed upon seeing her home so messy and disorganized and said that she thought her living environment was contributing to her depression. She said she felt she had no control of anything in her life. We collaboratively developed a plan to wash her dishes and put them in the cupboard and wash the clothes and organize them for use. Together we worked throughout the afternoon to complete these tasks and as we worked the client discussed her plans for the next day in which she intended to leave the hospital. She wanted to better organize her mail, to sort important mail from the junk so that she could pay her bills on time. As she reassumed control of her living situation, she was empowered to address other problems that had led to her hospitalization.

The Canadian Model of Occupational Performance places the client at the center of his environment. In this model of practice, the environment provides the opportunities and the challenges for living (Law & Mills, 1998; Baum, 1998). The client is influenced and motivated by physical, spiritual, affective and cognitive factors to perform valued occupations. Changes that the client experiences as a result of illness or injury result in a need to adapt to the environment through occupation. This process is dynamic; changes occur in the client and in the environment throughout the life span, as well as when illness or injury occur (Kielhofner, 2002). Community practice of occupational therapy can be naturally and rapidly responsive to changes in the client's environment or to the client's perceptions of self (Sumsion, 1999).

The focus of the International Classification of Impairment, Disability and Handicap is a model of functioning and disability in which performance is the central feature affected by health condition, environment, and personal factors. In this model, body function and structural impairments represent deviation from generally accepted population standards. These impairments may be temporary or permanent, but they do not automatically indicate that a person should be considered disabled. Participation in life tasks that integrate one into community illustrates the greater importance of function over disability. Function and performance of self-care, mobility, communication, learning, working, and interacting with others and the community are areas to be addressed by healthcare providers. Within the ICF model, contextual and personal factors, including the environment, interact with function and structure to either facilitate or constrain performance of the individual. Removing barriers and facilitating accessibility improves opportunities for performance within one's community (World Health Organization, 2001).

In order to view community practice as inclusive of different models and frameworks of practice, I propose an equation for viewing a client within the community. An occupational therapy practitioner will call upon her knowledge of and skills in a variety of evaluation and intervention strategies to engage in client centered community services.

Figure 2–1 illustrates this equation, with the person who is to perform valued functions relying on her human attributes as assets and/or constraints. Human attributes include spirit, cognition, affect, and physical condition (Sumsion, 1999) or other characteristics as identified in different practice models and frameworks. A person may have impairment in a particular attribute, but would be able to utilize other attributes to adapt and minimize or eliminate disability in functional performance in the community. Performance includes all of the functions that have purpose and meaning to the client, such as activities of daily living and instrumental activities of daily living, participation in work, leisure, and the social activities of the community.

PERFORMANCE = (Culture) +/- Environmental Factors +/- Human Attributes

Figure 2–1 What performance entails.

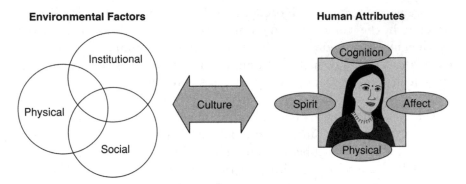

Figure 2–2 Interplay of environmental factors and human attributes.

Environmental factors of a community consist of physical, social, and institutional elements that facilitate or constrain optimal human performance. Conyne and Clack (1981) developed an environmental assessment model that identifies factors of the environment as either supporting or constraining satisfaction to those working or living in that environment. This model, illustrated in Figure 2-2, uses a Venn diagram of overlapping physical, social, and institutional factors. Within each area of the Venn diagram, environmental factors are identified as either constraints or assets to human function and satisfaction. Experience with this model has shown that most elements of the environment affecting performance fall into overlapping segments of the Venn diagram (Meyers, 1989). Therefore when using this model, one comes to understand that community environments to support performance require adaptation in multiple areas and that an occupational therapy practitioner must address these in order to remove constraints to performance. For example, observations in a particular community find that a lack of curb cuts significantly limits independent mobility of any person using a wheelchair. This barrier is a physical-institutional-social one because curb cuts physically help to increase social activities, but likely require a governmental directive to equalize access of community for all. In order to remedy this constraint, a therapist must advocate at the institutional level for funding of curb cuts, while at the same time working with planners to construct curb cuts that physically enable wheelchair mobility.

Environmental factors as well as human attributes are interpreted through a cultural lens. As Fitzgerald et al. (1997) reported, occupational therapy practitioners and their clients may not share cultures and as a result may interpret human problems and environmental factors differently.

Although culture is often evident in the roles and performance expected from an individual within a given culture, cultural values and beliefs have a broader implication for acceptance of therapy intervention. In community practice, the occupational therapy practitioner must strive to see the world through the client's cultural lens. Reflective of pre-theoretical reasoning, as described by Hooper (1997) in her discussion of assumptions that underlie clinical reasoning, these same pre-theoretical assumptions play a significant role in patterns of performance in one's own culture. These include the person's beliefs about reality, life, death and eternity, human nature, and the nature of knowing (Hooper, 1997). Each of these beliefs must be explored with a client in order to plan therapy that will be culturally acceptable.

As we conclude this section about client centered care in community practice, it may be beneficial to become aware of disability studies that examine physical, social, and institutional environmental factors that stigmatize and create barriers to inclusion for persons with disabilities. Generally these studies describe societal discriminatory factors regarding persons with physical and psychological disabilities, while at the same time advocating for the rights of persons with disabilities (Charleton, 1998). The focus is on empowerment of persons with disabilities to engage in whatever activities they find meaningful and satisfying by removing discriminatory barriers (Baylies, 2002). Voices of persons with physical and psychological disabilities offer valuable information that can be incorporated into practice. In my work with persons with severe and chronic mental illness, several of my clients advocated for their needs through participation in local government, writing for publication, and speaking in their communities. They wanted to be fully included in the activities of their communities, free to choose involvement in whatever productive or leisure activities appealed to them. Part of my work was to facilitate and support them in their efforts to be heard and included. Disability studies often bring clients, therapists, and other health providers together in their efforts to change perceptions of disabilities, to remove barriers, and to challenge the stereotypes that limit full access to living in inclusive communities.

CHAPTER SUMMARY

This chapter identified traditional elements of occupational therapy practice and re-framed them as they could be used in community practice. Temporal adaptation, support for clinical challenges, creative approaches to adaptive devices, and personal safety are often handled in unique ways outside of institutional environments. Awareness of one's own culture and becoming knowledgeable about other cultures are essential to establishing a therapeutic relationship with culturally diverse clients. Client centered practice, with special attention paid to environmental factors that influence success in achieving goals at home and in the community, provide the foundation for client success in adaptive performance.

LEARNING ACTIVITIES

Temporal Adaptation

Individuals approach and manage time in different ways; some prefer a schedule with deadlines prepared for them, and others like to plan for themselves. These are personal preferences that may influence job satisfaction and should be considered in choosing certain types of community practice.

Complete one of the following sentences:

1. I prefer to work where I have firmly established work hours, timelines for completion of projects, and where work time is separate from my personal time because . . .
2. I prefer to have flexible work hours so that I can set my own schedule, and complete work at home, because . . .

Some things to consider: scheduling abilities; procrastination; balance in work and leisure; multitasking

Challenge and Support

Camaraderie in the office can make work more enjoyable. Yet working in community practice often means working alone without other occupational therapy practitioners to share daily discussions. Preferences for working with others or working alone may change over time.

Complete one of the following sentences:

1. It would be difficult for me to work somewhere I did not have colleagues to interact with each day because . . .
2. I enjoy working alone and feel confident that the services I provide clients are excellent because . . .

Some things to consider: independence; gossip; finding mentors; using technology; need for reassurance

Autonomy

Some community practice is within organizations that provide structure for work. Solo practice or contractual work will need to be structured by the provider, who also will have responsibility for its outcomes. In choosing community practice where you would work alone, you will consider your attitudes toward working in a group and assuming responsibility.

Complete one of the following sentences:

1. I prefer to work where my work is structured by organization policies and procedures because . . .
2. I enjoy planning and organizing my own work and am comfortable being responsible for myself because . . .

Things to consider: response to authority; self-confidence; knowledge and skills; work ethic; responsibility

Personal Safety

Community practice, and addressing the issue of social justice, may at times involve going into a variety of areas and neighborhoods to provide services to clients in their homes. Navigating in unfamiliar areas, or being responsible for treating a client living in an area known to have criminal activity, can present a challenge.

Complete one of the following sentences:

1. I would find it difficult to go into a home to treat a client if she lived in an unsafe neighborhood because . . .
2. Concerns that I may have about going into an unsafe neighborhood to treat a client may addressed by . . .

Things to consider: safety precautions; social justice; the basis of fear; adaptability

Client Centered Care

Clients may be unaware that they are welcome participants in client centered health care decisions.

Many older adults continue to leave care decisions to professional providers as was customary in the past. How might you empower an older adult to participate in decisions related to the care you will be providing?

In some cultures, the role of decision-maker may be assigned according to age or gender. For example, a husband might make treatment decisions for a wife based on cultural expectations. How might you work with this couple to implement client centered care?

While planning home care services, clients may feel empowered to tell you what they want you to provide. If their desires conflict with what you are able to offer, or with what your professional judgment tells you would benefit them, how will you work toward an agreeable treatment program?

Exploring Community Context

Visit a community resource and focus on a space used by the public, such as a room in a library, a grocery store, or a swimming pool. Develop a Venn diagram, as illustrated in this chapter, of barriers to participation by a person using a wheelchair. Classify each barrier into physical, social, institutional, or overlapping areas. Describe how you would remove these barriers to participation. What challenges occur when barriers fall into overlapping areas such as physical-institutional or social-institutional-physical?

REFERENCES

Baum, C. (1998). Client-centered practice in a changing healthcare system. In: M. Law (Ed.) *Client-centered occupational therapy*. (pp. 29–46). Thorofare, NJ: Slack, Inc.

Baylies, C. (2002). Disability and the notion of human development: Questions of rights and capabilities. *Disability and society, 17* (7) 725–739.

Bonder, B., Martin, L. & Miracle, A.W. (2004). Culture emergent in occupation. *The American Journal of Occupational Therapy, 58* (2) 159–168.

Bourke-Taylor, H. & Hudson, D. (2005). Cultural differences: The experience of establishing an occupational therapy service in a developing community. *Australian Occupational Therapy Journal, 52,* 188–198.

Charleton, J. (1998). *Nothing about us without us.* Berkeley, CA: University of California Press.

Conyne, R.K. & Clack, J. (1981). *Environmental assessment and design: A new tool for the applied behavioral scientist.* New York: Praeger.

Crabtree, B.F. & Miller, W. (1998). *Doing qualitative research (2nd ed.)* Thousand Oaks, CA: Sage.

Creswell, J.W. (2007). *Qualitative inquiry and research design: Choosing among five approaches (2nd ed.)* Thousand Oaks, CA: Sage.

Fatehi, K. (2008). *Managing internationally: Succeeding in a culturally diverse world.* Thousand Oaks, CA: Sage.

Fitzgerald, M.H., Mullavey-O'Byrne, C. & Clemson, L. (1997). Cultural issues from practice. *Australian Occupational Therapy Journal, 44,* 1–21.

Folland, S., Goodman, A.C. & Stano, M. (2007). *The economics of health and health care (5th ed.)* Upper Saddle River, NJ: Prentice Hall.

Hesse-Biber, S.N. & Leavey, P. (2006). *The practice of qualitative research.* Thousand Oaks, CA: Sage.

Hooper, B. (1997). The relationship between pre-theoretical assumptions and clinical reasoning. *The American Journal of Occupational Therapy, 51* (5) 328–338.

Kielhofner, G. (2002). *A model of human occupation: Theory and application.* Baltimore, MD: Lippincott, Williams & Wilkins.

Kielhofner, G. (2004). *Conceptual foundations of occupational therapy (3rd ed.).* Philadelphia, PA: F.A. Davis.

Kielhofner, G. (1997). Temporal adaptation: A conceptual framework for occupational therapy. *The American Journal of Occupational Therapy, 31* (4) 236–242.

Law, M. & Mills, J. (1998). Client centered occupational therapy. In: M. Law (Ed.) *Client centered occupational therapy* (pp. 1–18). Thorofare, NJ: Slack, Inc.

Litterst, T.A.E. (1985). A reappraisal of anthropological fieldwork methods and the concept of culture in occupational therapy research. *The American Journal of Occupational Therapy, 39,* 602–604.

Meyers, S. (1989). Evaluation of occupational therapy level II fieldwork environments: A qualitative approach. *Occupational Therapy Journal of Research, 9* (6) 347–361.

Royeen, M. & Crabtree, J.L. (2006). *Culture in rehabilitation: From competency to proficiency.* Upper Saddle River, NJ: Pearson, Prentice Hall.

Scaffa, M. (2001). *Occupational therapy in community-based practice settings.* Philadelphia, PA: F.A. Davis.

Sumsion, T. (1999). *Client-centered practice in occupational therapy: A guide to implementation.* London: Churchill Livingstone

Tickle-Degnen, L. (2002). Evidence-based practice forum: Client-centered practice, therapeutic relationship and use of research evidence. *The American Journal of Occupational Therapy, 56* (4) 470–474.

World Health Organization (2001). *International classification of functioning, disability and health.* Geneva, Switzerland: World Health Organization.

II
Section

Exploring Developed Practice in the Community: Opportunities for Practice

Chapters 3 through 6 introduce community practices developed over the past 30 years. Each chapter describes community practice options including working with children and adolescents, adults, aging adults, and individuals with mental illness. Each chapter includes Stories from Practice as told by experienced therapists in order to give you a sense of some of the benefits and challenges of community practice. Though some of the types of community practices described in this section employ significant numbers of therapists, options for less familiar community practice areas are also identified.

If you are considering moving into the community to practice but are uncertain if this option is right for your needs, the practices described in these chapters may provide information that influences your decision. Most of the practice options presented are well established and offered through formal organizations that provide some job security in the form of a contract, a salary, or an established method for payment for your services. Many offer benefits important to therapists, such as health insurance and vacations. At the same time these practice options may offer flexibility in working hours and autonomy in work environment, both of which provide an incentive for many occupational therapy practitioners to move to community practice.

Chapter 3

Community Practice with Children and Adolescents

LEARNING OBJECTIVES

- Identify existing community practice options for children and adolescents.
- Create effective strategies for working with parents and teachers.
- Explain how occupational therapy helps address public health concerns of children and adolescents.

INTRODUCTION

This chapter will introduce you to some of the existing occupational therapy community practices with children. These practices provide occupational therapy practitioners interested in moving into community practice with varying levels of autonomy, offering either highly structured or, alternatively, more flexible work patterns. In the United States, schools provide the largest area of employment opportunity for occupational therapy practitioners (AOTA, 2007). In addition, occupational therapists join other rehabilitation professionals working with children who are under age three in community based early intervention programs for children with developmental delays. An emphasis on working with very young children became a government mandate with the acknowledgement that early intervention can decrease the number of services children with developmental delays will require as they grow older. Infants and preschool children are prepared to attend school with typically developing peers and perform at a higher level than if no therapy services were offered during their early development.

DEVELOPMENTAL ROLES AND CHALLENGES OF CHILDREN

The objective of rehabilitation services for school-age children is to facilitate learning and community integration. The goals of occupational therapy for children extend beyond the school years, however, into young adulthood with interventions designed to integrate a young adult into his community and its social, leisure, and work opportunities. Programs for children and adolescents are based on economic concerns to minimize costs of care, and on social justice by providing education for all children of all abilities. Children who receive early intervention may be less likely to require special services when they enter school, and children who receive education enhanced by special services are more likely to become independent adults and contribute to the national economy through employment.

When working with children in the community, an occupational therapy practitioner will work closely with parents and teachers as well as the child. This collaboration requires a different approach than one might experience in hospital based clinical practice. In the clinic the service provider is in control of her work environment. Parents or other caregivers bring the child to the clinic and the occupational therapy practitioner provides intervention and offers information that she determines will be helpful to the child and family. Working in the community, a service provider is either in the home environment of the child or the work environment of a teacher; in either situation, the occupational therapy practitioner no longer has complete control of her practice environment.

The parent of a child is responsible for both home and child, and this responsibility will largely determine the outcomes of occupational therapy either directly or indirectly. If a parent does not feel that a service provider is supportive of her needs or helpful to her child, the parent may decide not continue with therapy sessions. The parent may cancel or just not be home when the service provider arrives. If an occupational therapy practitioner fails to understand the parent's needs as well as the child's needs, she will have a difficult if not impossible task in getting the parent to comply with her recommendations. Using client centered care in which children, parents, or caregivers are at the center of service decisions is an important approach to community based occupational therapy for children.

Teachers are in charge of their classrooms and are held accountable for academic performance of their pupils. Just like parents, they are busy with their responsibility to teach children and to raise scores on nationally mandated education tests. If an occupational therapy practitioner cannot make the teacher's job of teaching more effective, a teacher may see her as a distraction or, worse, a nuisance in the classroom. Collaborating with teachers is an important part of the school based practice of occupational therapy.

PRACTICE IN EARLY INTERVENTION PROGRAMS

Early intervention provides services to children up to age three in order to enhance a child's development in a natural environment (Stephens & Tauber, 2005). In the United States, Part C of the *Individuals with Disabilities Act* supports individual states to provide comprehensive services to each child, birth to age three, with an environmental or biological risk of developmental delay (IDEA, 2004). The services provided to these children are designed to be multidisciplinary and include occupational therapy, speech therapy, physical therapy, nursing, education, and other services as needed to address developmental delays in the very young child. Children referred for evaluation are assigned a service coordinator who is responsible for the child's evaluation and assists the family in accessing information and service providers determined by evaluation as necessary to enhance the child's development (IDEA, 1997). Early intervention services must be provided in the child's natural environment. Therefore most children in this age group are evaluated and provided with intervention at home, although some children may be seen in daycare programs or other locations that are part of their natural environment in the community.

Providing occupational therapy to children in the community offers opportunities and challenges to a practitioner. In a medical clinic setting, an occupational therapy practitioner must rely on a parent's report to try to understand what home life is like for a child. Young children learn from their environments, developing through sensory stimulation, social interactions with others, and by managing challenging activities or obstacles. In the child's home, the occupational therapy practitioner has an opportunity to observe these phenomena and use them to guide intervention. Once she enters a child's home, the occupational therapy practitioner can experience for herself noise or other distractions that exist in the environment. Stimuli that may seem unremarkable to a parent familiar with the environment may be identified by a therapist as overwhelming for a child. In home practice, a service provider observes how the child is integrated into family life, how the child interacts with siblings, what type of play is allowed or encouraged, and the contributions a child makes to others in the family.

A Story from Practice

While working in the community with an adult client, I had an opportunity to observe a four-month-old infant who had spent her first two months of life in the hospital. When this little girl came home from the hospital she was still receiving oxygen. During visits to her home, I observed that she was always in a reclining plastic baby seat in the middle of the family's living room. As I talked with my client, I asked her and other family members in the home if they ever moved the baby from this particular seat. They all replied that she was indeed always in this baby seat except for diaper or clothing changes. When she cried or fussed, she was immediately fed. Although this baby was usually surrounded by her playing siblings, they were instructed never to touch her. The child's mother reliably took her baby to her scheduled clinic visits and the baby's physical health continued to improve; in fact her weight increased more than expected. She began, however, to experience developmental delays that the clinic attributed to her low birth weight. One of the goals of my intervention with the baby's mother was to support her parenting role. Thus the clinic contacted me when they became concerned about the infant's significant weight gain. This gave me an opportunity to discuss with my client the possibility of having some additional services to facilitate her baby's development. It would take a few months to implement these additional services. In the meantime, I was asked to provide information to the mother about development of premature infants and the need to move her little girl from her baby seat to other positions in order to stimulate development of head and neck control and to improve her strength. The child's environmental barriers to development began to be removed, and she began to develop motor and social skills through interaction with her brothers and sisters. Without observation of the child in her home, the environmental barriers contributing to her developmental delay might have gone undetected for some time.

An occupational therapy practitioner working in early intervention will focus on a child's development of adaptive behavior and play as well as sensory-motor and postural development. The practitioner may facilitate an adaptive environment and may provide assistive or orthotic devises to facilitate further development and acquisition of functional skills (Stephens & Tauber, 2005). Early intervention evaluation is functional when it focuses on the child's need and ability to relate and adapt to her environment. Evaluations used with the birth-to-age-three population are the same as those used in clinic environments. An occupational therapy practitioner working in a child's home, however, will also have the opportunity to evaluate the natural environment of the child. She may observe the child in her home while asking questions about the types of activities in which the child engages. The occupational therapy practitioner can see physical or social barriers that may influence the child's participation in family life. Using analytical skills, an occupational therapy practitioner can remove barriers that delay development, or help to facilitate a child's participation in family life. Evaluation is an ongoing process in response to continual changes in the child and the child's environments.

Intervention for children at home involves a child's family or other caregivers. Working with a developmentally delayed young child involves special challenges. Wooster (2001) identifies mothers who care for disabled children to be at risk for social isolation. Additionally, some families with disabled children live in economically disadvantaged communities and are unable to purchase toys or provide other developmentally enriching experiences for their children. This does not imply that a financially disadvantaged mother is less interested in her child's development than a mother with more economic resources. She may be aware of activities that would enhance her child's development but be unable to afford these toys or experiences. Additional stressors to families with a developmentally delayed child may include being a household headed by a single parent, or dysfunction in family interactions due to a parent with mental illness, substance abuse, or social deprivation. Even when families are not economically or otherwise disadvantaged, however, the care of a child with disabilities places significant strain on the caregiver (Crowe & Florez, 2006).

Partnerships or marriages often do not survive the arrival of a disabled child. For several years, a group of therapists has annually visited a country without benefit of occupational therapy services, where the majority of children who receive therapy are in homes headed by a single parent. The usual story is that the father left the family when the child was identified as having a disability, placing full responsibility to care for the child on the mother or grandmother. Olson and Esdaile (2000) studied mothers of children diagnosed with cerebral palsy. These mothers described living in "survival" mode. Their lives consisted primarily of providing physical care and nurturing for their disabled children while trying to advocate for their children's needs. It is recognized that parenting a child with a disability is difficult and lonely and that support helps the parent to cope, but this support is often minimal or lacking.

VanLeit and Crowe (2002) proposed the need for occupational therapy practitioners to provide family centered care as opposed to intervention for just the child with developmental delay or disability. The family is responsible for the child and his care, and through learning and continuing to implement techniques introduced by the occupational therapy practitioner, the family can be a change agent for the child. Parents can also be empowered to act as the child's advocate throughout life (Stephens & Tauber, 2005). Unless an occupational therapy practitioner focuses on the entire family, her influence in the child's development may have limited value.

Understanding the role of parenting a child with a disability is important in establishing a therapeutic relationship. Mothering is a complex blend of planning, organizing, interpreting, anticipating, predicting, and understanding what is needed to care for a child. Most of these tasks are complex cognitive activities that require multitasking. The role of mothering also requires flexibility in managing the family and the home, and skill in delegating to others (Richardson, 2002). Recognizing that her child has a disability, coping with options of intervention, strained family relationships, and changes in economic status as a result of job loss or the cost of health care can all challenge cognitive functions and make mothering more difficult.

A Story from Practice

A mother of a child with a disability is a therapist and knows that her child needs additional attention to facilitate his development. Even with her knowledge, she often feels overwhelmed by the time and energy needed for activities to maximize her child's development. This mother has an advantage, however, that other mothers may not have; as a therapist she knows what services are available and how to obtain these services for her child. By being able to delegate to others some of her child's care, she is able to reduce the stress on her life that comes from mothering a child with a disability. Knowing how to navigate a system of services available, but not necessarily easy to obtain, is an advantage in reducing this mother's feelings of frustration. Most parents do not have this mother's knowledge or skills and bear a great burden of care alone.

When working with children in the community, the occupational therapy practitioner must know which services are available to children and their families and how to access them. She rarely can provide a family with everything they need to parent a child with a disability, but she can put parents in touch with other resources to decrease the burden of parenting.

In order to address a parent's needs in caring for a developmentally disabled child at home, an occupational therapy practitioner might use the Canadian Occupational Performance Measure to initiate a conversation with the mother about her roles and performance (Law et al., 1998). Using this instrument can help introduce discussion about tasks of mothering as well as satisfaction or frustration associated with those tasks. Such discussion allows the occupational therapy practitioner to collaborate with the mother in providing care for her child while also caring for the mother's needs. The mother becomes an active participant in her child's therapy when she feels comfortable enough to ask questions and receive information that will allow her to make decisions about her child's care. An occupational therapy practitioner needs to be nonjudgmental in listening to a mother's frustrations about her roles and responsibilities, so that together mother and therapist can establish a therapeutic relationship that benefits the child as well as all other members of the child's family.

Working in the community environment, an occupational therapy practitioner must be flexible about scheduling to meet the parents' and child's needs. She must be able to modify intervention plans to respond to changes in the child or his environment. The tools for intervention may be found in everyday activities of a child's life; an occupational therapy practitioner may use toys that she brings to the child's home, but more often she uses the toys or other playthings already available in the home. She may suggest toys or play opportunities available within the community that would enhance a child's development. Being familiar with community resources is an advantage in making treatment recommendations to parents. Knowing where safe play equipment is available for young children at local sites such as parks or museums can help the occupational therapy practitioner specifically direct the child's family to the most satisfying play options. By referring parents to community programs offered for preschool-age children, and specifying their locations and costs, an occupational therapy practitioner can enhance a child's development beyond what can be provided through time-limited intervention sessions. Some community programs provide play opportunities for young children in tandem with social opportunities and support for parents, thereby meeting the therapeutic needs of both mother and child.

SCHOOL-BASED PRACTICE

Occupational therapy in schools is designed to facilitate a child's ability to learn through inclusion in a general education curriculum (IDEA, 2004). Schools are required to provide therapy for those children whose disabilities may interfere with their learning (Case-Smith & Rogers, 2005). Schools provide therapy services in various ways: Some schools hire their own therapists, other schools have contractual arrangements with agencies to provide therapy services, or schools may contract directly with therapists who are self-employed. Therapy interventions also vary from one school jurisdiction to another and are often determined by parent demand balanced against school budget constraints.

School-based occupational therapy practitioners have traditionally responded by providing services when parents, teachers, or school administrators have identified children unable to acquire or master skills required for satisfactory school performance. Children of all abilities attend school, including some with mobility challenges. Teaching a child how to access and utilize school facilities enhances performance in activities of daily living and increases social participation, both of which may improve academic performance (Case-Smith, 2005). A recent trend calls for children to be referred to an occupational therapy practitioner for handwriting, because illegible writing interferes with academic performance and outcomes testing. Most teachers have little preparation for teaching handwriting and rarely have expertise in teaching handwriting to children with sensory perception or motor skill challenges. In addition, little time is available in the curriculum to teach handwriting skills, prompting teachers to refer children with difficulty in handwriting to an occupational therapy practitioner (Donica, 2008). The majority of children, however, who are believed to benefit from occupational therapy in the schools have sensory-perception, motor and praxis, cognitive, or social skill disabilities that interfere with social participation and education. An estimated 20 percent of children and adolescents have a disabling mental health condition (Belfer, 2008). Many children are referred to an occupational therapy practitioner when their classroom behavior is disruptive and a teacher has difficulty managing their education process. (Case-Smith & Rogers, 2005).

One example is children with attention deficit hyperactivity disorder (ADHD) who may disrupt a teacher's activities and distract their classmates. These children may move about in their chairs or talk when they should be quiet and attentive. Some of these children appear to be disinterested in what is being presented by the teacher to the extent that some may fall asleep in class. These distracting behaviors exhibited by a child create a difficult learning environment for the majority of students in the class. This can lead to classroom management problems for a teacher who may then ask an occupational therapy practitioner to intervene with the disruptive child. An occupational therapy practitioner may provide intervention in adaptive strategies for the child or the teacher to improve the child's school performance. An economic concern to society arises when more than one-half of all children with a diagnosis of ADHD drop out of school, mainly because they experience social difficulties and poor academic performance that lead to cycles of failure and poor self-esteem. These children are intellectually able to perform academic work, but they have difficulty responding and adapting to sensory information coming from the environment. Most of these children find themselves in environments that are over-stimulating or under-stimulating and their brains cannot make meaning of what they see, hear, smell, or feel (Parham & Mailloux, 2005).

Therapy for some children with sensory processing disorders has resulted in removing them from their classrooms for therapy or special help with learning. While this type of treatment has benefited the child by allowing him to focus on specific learning tasks without bombardment of sensory information in the classroom environment, it identifies the child as "different" from the other children in his class. This creates doubt in the child's image of himself at an age when fitting in and being like other children is important. Although removing a child from the classroom may address the problem temporarily, the child must soon return to a classroom filled with the same sensory distractions. Treatment within the classroom, on the other hand, provides the advantage of potentially modifying the natural learning environment to be less distracting for all children. It may also more effectively enhance a child's self-image, as he is not singled out as being disruptive and different from his peers.

In order to provide effective intervention in a classroom environment a teacher may collaborate with an occupational therapy practitioner (Bose & Hinojosa, 2008). While some teachers have an understanding of occupational therapy intervention to enhance a child's performance in learning, other teachers will just be discovering the many contributions that an occupational therapy practitioner can make to students in a school environment. Any time an occupational therapy practitioner is given an opportunity to explain occupational therapy to another person, she must carefully examine her own motivation and methods for explaining her services. Teachers, as well as other potential collaborators, do not appreciate being told that there is something important they do not know. This creates an unequal relationship between teacher and therapist and interferes with successful collaboration (Bose & Hinojosa, 2008). An occupational therapy practitioner must take the initiative to discover a teacher's goals for her own performance of her role as teacher. With this knowledge, the practitioner can provide information to assist the teacher toward her goals and at the same time invite collaboration in assisting children to maximize their performance in the classroom. Children who are disruptive or present classroom management problems are a concern for most teachers. Beginning a discussion around these behaviors, and proposing intervention that is inclusive of all children, provides an ideal opportunity to engage a teacher in a discussion about the needs of children with disabilities.

Finding common interests is important to collaboration. Teachers and occupational therapy practitioners both are concerned with the development of children in their care, which provides a common language for discussing how to help a child socially develop within a classroom environment. As collaborators, teacher and therapist can construct an environment that maximizes competency of all children in the classroom, regardless of whether or not they are children with disabilities. When a therapist helps solve classroom management problems and enhances performance of children, she becomes a valuable collaborator and a continuing resource for the teacher and her students.

Although some children respond best to intervention outside the classroom that is focused on specific strategies for organizing their work and enhancing academic performance, therapists may have more significant impact on an entire group of children by providing treatment in the classroom. An example provided by Schilling et al. (2003) reports results of an occupational therapy program for children with ADHD that included all children in a classroom, both those with ADHD and those without the diagnosis. The therapist introduced therapy balls in place of chairs for all children in a classroom. The therapy balls were determined to increase attention and performance for all children in classroom activities. The results indicated that attending behavior and legible word production in written work improved for children with ADHD. All of the children in the class thought the balls increased their seating comfort, improved their handwriting and ability to listen to the teacher, and to complete their work. One child with ADHD reported that a disadvantage of using a therapy ball as a seat was that he could not sleep in class when he had to sit on the ball. Although the child considered this a disadvantage, any child needs to be awake in order to learn, thereby making this "disadvantage" a positive outcome of the therapist's intervention.

A Story from Practice

While working with children with ADHD in a clinic setting, we found that these children responded well to the ALERT therapy program in which children identify their level of attention and then choose "tools" to maintain their attention at an optimal level (Williams & Shellenberger, 1994). Some of the tools that children could choose included objects to manipulate with their hands; food or chewing gum for their oral motor needs; or therapy balls for seating. While these tools worked well in the clinic, most of them were not allowed in the classroom—where these children's behaviors were most disruptive. In order to take this intervention to an environment where it would have more substantial effect, we engaged teachers in understanding ADHD as a sensory modulation problem. The teachers learned that children could identify when they were having difficulty and could choose tools to improve their behavior in the classroom. Teachers were given opportunities to select tools that they found helpful in reducing their own stress or anxiety and through this experience began to understand how this could help children in their classrooms. This realization led to the introduction of the ALERT program to an

> *entire classroom including children with and without ADHD. Each child, along with the teacher, discovered which tools worked best to help them maintain optimal arousal. As the tools were used in the classroom, all the children enjoyed the benefits of improved behavior and performance.*

COMMUNITY SERVICES FOR OLDER CHILDREN WITH PHYSICAL DISABILITIES

Some children with physical disabilities have been found to have impaired social development at home and at school. Richardson (2002) described a cycle of limited environmental engagement opportunities leading to social, emotional, and psychological disabilities that persisted into adulthood for children with physical disabilities. As adults, these individuals experience isolation, poor self-esteem, poor social adjustment, and diminished employment. Schools, in which children form social units that may be exclusionary, were identified as contributing to the barriers these children experienced with social integration. Families were also found to contribute to these problems because parents or other family members tended to compensate for social and other environmental problems so that the child learned to turn to adults or helpful peers when an obstacle appeared. When socialization with peers was not satisfactory, children with disabilities missed opportunities to master the challenges of social relationships, a tendency which persisted into adulthood.

Richardson's (2002) study illustrates how children with physical disabilities engage in play or social interactions that focus on themselves when they are shunned by peers, or move from one group of peers to another, unable to sustain involvement in one group over time. As a result, they did not seem to learn or understand the importance of reciprocity in peer relationships (Richardson, 2002). Because of the importance of social integration to life satisfaction in adulthood, many children with physical disabilities must be taught to engage in reciprocal interactions with non-disabled peers. Occupational therapy practitioners, with their knowledge of physical, cognitive, and psychological development, as well as their understanding of the effects of disabling conditions on a person's ability to perform in context, may facilitate social integration through community involvement. As children with impairments in performance skills graduate from public education programs where they may have received services specified by the *Individuals with Disabilities Act* (IDEA, 2004), there are opportunities in community practice for occupational therapy practitioners to offer services to integrate these children into employment and social participation.

Fazio (2008) identifies many full-time, part-time, or voluntary options to provide occupational therapy in community settings. Therapists have long been engaged in participating in camping programs for children of all ages with disabilities. There are many camps that have been developed to serve children with specific healthcare needs, such as camps for children with cancer or burns, or for children who are wheelchair users or who are ventilator dependent. These camps value contributions made by occupational therapy practitioners and students providing children with experiences to enhance their sense of self, acquisition of social skills, and age appropriate fun. Community organizations sponsor clubs such as scouting or sports and recreation programs that are inclusive of persons with disabilities. University students enrolled in health profession degree programs often participate in these types of experiences as part-time or summer employees, or as part of their clinical education experience. Many students continue their involvement in these programs into their professional careers. Special Olympics, an organization that offers children and adults opportunities to learn sports and compete among their peers, values therapists' involvement in its programs. Sharing their love of a sport, teaching it to others, and coaching in games at local, national, and international levels, are ways therapists contribute their skills to their communities. Unlimited opportunities exist for therapists to volunteer within their communities and work with children and adolescents with disabilities in dance, music, and other arts, and sports and recreation. Utilizing talents and leisure preferences as a community volunteer may eventually lead to acquiring part-time or full-time employment that unites personal interests with your professional skills and knowledge and proves especially fulfilling.

COMMUNITY PRACTICE RELATED TO DEVELOPMENTAL CHALLENGES OF ADOLESCENTS

Many opportunities likewise exist for occupational therapy practitioner to provide community services for adolescents with and without disabilities. Adolescents are in a period of transition in which they are assessing personal strengths or abilities and attempting to find their future direction by matching their assets and challenges with community opportunities. The direction that an adolescent takes in his life is determined by people and opportunities in his environment. One task of adolescence is to prepare for a productive work life. Some adolescents will be influenced by family expectations to pursue a specific type of work or a university education to prepare for a career. Some adolescents do not have family support for choosing their future directions; they may instead be influenced by teachers or others significant in their lives. Some adolescents, limited in their options for further education or work life by intellectual disabilities or socioeconomic factors, will need direction to find satisfying work consistent with their abilities. Although most adolescents successfully transition to adult life, there are some who do not. Social, physical, cognitive, and economic disadvantages may make it very difficult to prepare for a productive and satisfying adulthood that includes finding and keeping gainful employment.

Adolescents must also learn to establish interpersonal relationships with others of both genders. Social relationships provide a sense of belonging to a group and community and ease transition into work life. Engagement in social relationships stimulates involvement with others in leisure and service activities, which enriches a community. Direct relationships with others in one's community also provide support in times of challenge or stress. For most people, late adolescence begins a period of social interaction directed toward a search for a partner with whom to share life. Ideally, this partnership is one of mutual respect, caring, and support that endures throughout difficult periods of adulthood. These tasks of adolescents require the ability to learn, to plan, to take risks, and to maintain a sense of well-being. By utilizing their knowledge and skill, and providing services that can address intellectual and social challenges as well as economic disadvantages, occupational therapy practitioners facilitate adolescent development and help adolescents transition into satisfying adult roles in the community.

Ko and McEnery (2004) described an occupational therapy program for adolescents with physical disabilities engaged in transition to adult roles. These authors identified how the usual transition from school to adult living is more difficult for adolescents with physical disabilities. These adolescents were said to be less mature than their non-disabled peers, and some were less able to solve problems and make decisions related to transition to adult roles and responsibilities. Many adolescents with physical disabilities have fewer financial resources and opportunities for work and leisure than their non-disabled peers. At the same time they were transitioning from school to work or other productive activities, these adolescents lost their long-term relationships with children's services for rehabilitation and health care. The authors suggest that planning for these transitions should begin well before graduation or any other transitional period. Occupational therapy practitioners can address these transition challenges by empowering adolescents to advocate for their own physical and social needs. Therapists can introduce housing options independent of families and teach adolescents how to access transportation. They can facilitate selection of productive work consistent with a person's interests and abilities and teach skills required to secure employment. All of these services can be provided within the community where the adolescent lives and where he will work to achieve greater confidence in his abilities and the independence needed to pursue dreams.

Learning in one's own community environment has advantages. One advantage is that any obstacles to performance may be indentified, confronted, and overcome in a supportive environment before they must be done independently. This improves the learner's confidence that he can solve problems and manage activities that are necessary for daily occupational performance. For example, riding a bus can involve many complex skills such as reading and understanding bus schedules and bus routes. For a person with a disability, being able to ask for help and directions requires communication skills.

A Story from Practice

While I was riding a bus, it stopped for a young man who was using a wheelchair. The bus was equipped with a lift that should have lowered to the curb so that the man could direct his wheelchair onto the bus and manage his own transportation. On this particular day, the lift on the bus refused to work. It would not lower to the curb. The bus driver, perhaps more concerned about his schedule than this young man's transportation, hastily told this young man to wait for the next bus. The man in the wheelchair, however, was not about to be inconvenienced by an equipment failure. He assertively instructed the bus driver on different strategies to try to get the lift to work. Eventually the lift lowered to the curb and the man got on the bus. He told the bus driver to call ahead and alert the bus company that the lift was not functioning properly, which the bus driver did.

As I observed this event, I realized that this young man using a wheelchair was highly skilled and knowledgeable. He knew how the lift worked, could give the driver instructions to make the lift operate, and was assertive in his communication. He was not going to let the bus driver leave him behind nor was he going to let the dysfunctional bus go unreported. Not everyone has the interest or ability to explain how to make a lift work, but all of our clients can be taught to be assertive so that their rights as community members are honored.

Adolescence can be a time of significant stress. Part of this is due to physical changes in the body, but stress also originates from the changes in routines, school and work environments, and social relationships that occur throughout the adolescent period. Occupational therapy practitioners continue to work with children with special needs in the schools throughout adolescence. Focusing on social and cognitive skills needed for work may become the focus of school based therapy for older children through their remaining school years. Transitioning to employment through part-time work, in which most older adolescents participate, may be facilitated for those with disabilities by working collaboratively with parents and potential employers. Assisting parents to understand how they can help their children navigate the transition from a relatively sheltered environment of school to the greater independence of adulthood is often overlooked and is an area where therapists working in the community can contribute. Occupational therapy practitioners may work with potential employers of adolescents to match worker skills with workplace demands. Occupational therapy practitioners can provide a valuable service by working with adolescents through community agencies to identify stressors and develop coping strategies. Volunteer opportunities abound for therapists who are welcomed into community organizations to help design and implement activities specifically for adolescents with differing abilities. Inclusion in community activities that can transition into adult leisure participation is important for all adolescents.

ADDRESSING LIFESTYLE CHALLENGES IN CHILDREN AND ADOLESCENTS

Occupational therapy practitioners working with children, adolescents, and young adults in the community have opportunities to address some of the challenges that unhealthy lifestyles have created. Specific health threats to young people arising from their environment include obesity, which can lead to cardiovascular disease, diabetes, and joint damage; substance abuse; and early sexual activity. Poulson and Ziviani (2004) identified ill health resulting from lifestyles of children as an economic concern to society. Many children have adopted a lifestyle that includes eating foods high in fat and sugar, and have become increasingly sedentary as they swap physical activity for computer games or television. These children are growing into overweight and unhealthy adolescents and adults. That obesity contributes to some of the costliest long-term illnesses of adulthood is an acknowledged fact (Folland, Stano & Goodman, 2007). Occupational therapy's holistic approach to intervention may therefore be able to contribute to a better understanding of why unhealthy lifestyle occurs and collaborate in discovering and providing remedies to these health concerns. Therapists can address the interpersonal, intrapersonal, and temporal aspects of occupational performance that influence obesity (Poulson & Ziviani, 2004). Occupational therapy practitioners can collaborate in community programs that serve children and adolescents by providing skills for living that combine an understanding of physical and mental health with disease prevention. Rather than being strictly informational, these programs would include active engagement in occupations that are meaningful and pleasurable to children and adolescents. Rather than learning about proper nutrition through a lecture or a book, an occupational therapy practitioner would provide active engagement of children in planning and preparing a meal that is healthy and tasty. Rather than talking about exercise, therapists would engage children in non-competitive games or sports, martial arts, or yoga that would be enjoyable. Whatever is offered to children must be interesting enough to compel them to leave their computers and televisions and give up tasty but unhealthy food. If options offered for healthy living are not appealing to children and adolescents, they will not listen nor act to improve their own health. Active learning allows occupational therapy to have its greatest impact on quality of life for the persons we serve.

CHAPTER SUMMARY

There are many children and adolescents in our communities who find aspects of their lives challenging. Some of these children receive occupational therapy, but the vast majority do not. Many opportunities exist for occupational therapy practitioners to develop and provide programs to enhance the quality of life for children and adolescents. The added benefit is that occupational therapy services can prevent future problems, lead to a more productive and satisfying adulthood, and reduce the need for costlier health care later in life. The community programs described in this chapter are only a few examples of existing opportunities for occupational therapy practitioners to utilize their skills and knowledge. There are many more opportunities for those who enjoy working with children and adolescents to engage in community practice.

LEARNING ACTIVITIES

Community practice may be designed to meet the needs and desires of people of all ages and abilities. This chapter, focused on the needs of children and their caregivers, provided some examples of community practice opportunities. Additional needs for occupational therapy services may be identified through the activities and questions provided.

1. Make a list of developmental tasks for a specific age range of childhood. From a perspective of life-span development, identify tasks of infants, preschoolers, elementary, middle, or high-school-age children, or older adolescents.
2. Identify barriers to participation in the developmental tasks you identified for this age group.

3. Consider why caregivers' wants and needs are important to any community practice.

4. What are some of the wants or needs of caregivers of the age of children you choose to describe in Question #1? You may want to interview a caregiver who has a child in the age range you have selected to find out what the caregiver wants for his or her child.

5. Having identified needs, wants, and expectations, if you were to develop a community program for children in this age range, what types of specific services would you provide?

6. What knowledge and special skills would you need if you were to develop and offer this program?

7. Locate and visit a program in your community that is similar to the program you described in Question #5. If you are unable to find a similar program, visit another community service for the age range you are exploring.
   • During your visit, observe children engaged in activity and note different abilities to engage and perform.
   • Observe barriers that exist for some children to perform the activities.
   • What could be done to remove these barriers?

8. Increasing knowledge of your community and problems that affect children and adolescents may lead to development of an occupational therapy practice or volunteer opportunity to address these problems. Find an article or story from your local news media that identifies a collective issue for children (e.g., obesity, inactivity, or homelessness) in your community. Develop a description of how an occupational therapy practitioner or occupational therapy program can address this community need.

REFERENCES

American Occupational Therapy Association (2007, July 30). 2006 Workforce and compensation survey: Occupational therapy salaries and job opportunities continue to improve. *OT Practice online*. Retrieved June 8, 2008 from http://aota.org/Pubs.

Belfer, M.L. (2008). Child and adolescent mental disorders: The magnitude of the problem around the globe. *Journal of Child Psychology and Psychiatry, 49* (3) 226–236.

Bose, P. & Hinojosa, J. (2008). Reported experiences from occupational therapists interacting with teachers in inclusive early childhood classrooms. *American Journal of Occupational Therapy, 62* (3) 289–297.

Case Smith, J. (Ed.) (2005). *Occupational therapy for children*. St. Louis, MO: Elsevier Mosby.

Case-Smith, J. & Rogers, J. (2005). School based occupational therapy (2nd ed.) In J. Case-Smith (Ed.) *Occupational therapy for children (5th ed., pp. 795–826).* St. Louis, MO: Elsevier Mosby.

Crowe, T.K. & Florez, S.J. (2006). Time use of mothers with school-age children: A continuing impact of a child's disability. *American Journal of Occupational Therapy, 60* (2) 194–203.

Donica, D. (2008). *An historical journey through the development of handwriting instruction.* Unpublished manuscript.

Fazio, L. (2008). *Developing occupation-centered programs for the community (2nd ed.).* Upper Saddle River, NJ: Pearson Prentice Hall.

Folland, S., Goodman, A.C. & Stano, M. (2007). *The economics of health care (5th ed.)* Upper Saddle River, NJ: Prentice Hall.

Individuals with Disabilities Act of 2004 Amendments. (P.L. 108–446). Retrieved January 18, 2009 from http://www.nichcy.org/Laws/IDEA/Pages/Buildingthelegacy.aspx *Individuals with Disabilities Education Act of 1997 Amendments.* (P.L. 105–17), 20 USC et seq.

Ko, B. & McEnery, G. (2004). The needs of physically disabled young people during transition to adult services. *Child: Care and Health Development, 30* (4) 317–323.

Law, M., Baptiste, S. Carswell, A., Polatajko, H. & Pollock, H. (1998). *The Canadian occupational performance measure (3rd ed.).* Toronto: CAOT Publications ACE.

Olson, J. & Esdaile, S. (2000). Mothering young children with disabilities in a challenging urban environment. *The American Journal of Occupational Therapy, 40,* 125–129.

Parham, L.D. & Mailloux, Z. (2005). Sensory integration. In: J. Case Smith (Ed.) *Occupational therapy for children (5th ed., pp. 356–409).* St. Louis, MO: Elsevier Mosby.

Poulson, A.A. & Ziviani, J.M. (2004). Health enhancing physical activity: Factors influencing engagement patterns in children. *Australian Occupational Therapy Journal, 51* 69–79.

Richardson, P. (2002). The school as social context: Social interaction patterns of children with physical disabilities. *American Journal of Occupational Therapy, 56* (3) 296–304.

Schilling, D.L., Washington, K., Billingsley, F.F. & Dietz, J. (2003). Classroom seating for children with attention deficit hyperactivity disorder: Therapy balls versus chairs. *American Journal of Occupational Therapy, 57* (5) 534–541.

Stephens, L.C. & Tauber, S.K. (2005). Early intervention. In J. Case Smith (Ed.) *Occupational therapy for children (5th ed., pp. 771–794).* St. Louis: MO; Elsevier Mosby.

VanLeit, B. & Crowe, T.K. (2002). Outcomes of an occupational therapy program for mothers of children with disabilities. *American Journal of Occupational Therapy, 56* (4) 402–410.

Williams, M.S. & Shellenberger, S. (1994). *How does your engine run? A leader's guide to the ALERT program for self-regulation.* Albuquerque NM: Therapy Works.

Wooster, D.A. (2001). Early intervention programs. In M. Scaffa (Ed.) *Occupational therapy in community-based practice settings.* (pp. 271–290). Philadelphia, PA: F.A. Davis Co.

Chapter 4

Community Practice
with Adults

- Identify performance skills and patterns of adults that would be enhanced by community services.
- Generate potential community practices for adults.
- Relate community practice with adults to economic conditions.

DEVELOPMENTAL ROLES AND CHALLENGES OF ADULTS

Physical Development

Adulthood is characterized by a continuum of changes that occur across a span of about 50 years. Early in their lives, young adults reach their maximum physical potential, which then begins a gradual decline over the duration of their remaining life spans. Capacity for physical performance varies throughout adulthood, however, as a result of a person's activity level, satisfaction with life, and experience of illness or injury. For many adults, physical health contributes to their well-being as it permits them to perform meaningful work and leisure activities.

Economic Development

Economic productivity is of significant concern throughout adulthood. Financial independence is usually achieved in early adulthood and continues throughout the life span. For most adults, there is an increase in economic status sometime in mid-adulthood that may extend until the time of retirement or may diminish over this same period. Reaching and maintaining financial stability has become a challenge for many people because of workplace adjustments and changes in response to shifts in national and world economies. In the past, the average worker could expect lifetime employment in the same job with the same employer, a situation which is no longer the norm for the majority of workers. Most adults today can expect to have numerous jobs with different employers throughout their lives (Peters, 2005). Some of these changes are a worker's choice, but more result from economic pressures beyond the worker's control. Health problems or disability, as well as environmental changes or events, may disrupt work patterns for adults.

Job loss due to local or national economic pressures leads to stress for the unemployed person coping with decreased or absent income and loss of his or her role as a worker. Changes that benefit an industry or an employer may not be good for affected workers and their families. A person who loses a job is challenged to find another job—one that may pay less than is needed to support himself and his family. Many types of jobs, such as those in manufacturing, have ceased to exist due to changes in technology. Some jobs have shifted to locations where production costs are lower. Other jobs are affected by decreased demand for goods and services. Periods of unemployment have increased as the national economy has declined; some lost industrial and manufacturing jobs may never return. Often, unemployed workers must be re-trained or relocate to find other jobs. Some displaced workers return to school to learn new skills in hopes of working in a different industry.

Job insecurity has led to role changes in families. A wife may need to support her family while her husband seeks a new job and assumes more home management responsibilities. Role strain is widespread due to many families who need both parents to work full time to support the family while also caring for children and the home. All of these events unfold in an economic environment that appears unreliable. In addition to environmental uncertainty, many families include one or more adults who work full time and may work multiple jobs, but still have difficulty rising above the poverty level. Economics plays a large role in life satisfaction for adults.

Family Life

Transitions related to family life occur throughout adulthood. Most young people find a partner and leave their parents to establish their own home. When beginning this partnership, both partners may work full time as they strive to establish themselves in their work or careers. Their employment role is the main focus of personal identity during this period. Young adults typically work long hours to establish their place in a career. Some return to school for another degree or specialized training to have better work opportunities in the future. Any of these time-intensive, productive activities may place strains on partner relationships.

At some point in early to middle adulthood, couples may choose to have children. Childbearing years are biologically limited, so this decision arises at a time when many prospective parents are thoroughly engaged in their careers. When a couple makes the decision to have a child, additional stress may occur; keep in mind that stress may result from any change, including positive experiences. Infertility has become an expensive and sometimes disappointing experience for couples, as technology boosts hope and then fails to meet expectations. Once a child is born, different stressors may appear for parents. One parent may stop working to care for the child, placing additional financial responsibility on the parent who continues to work to support the entire family. A parent who stays home to care for a child may experience a loss of work identity, which may lead to frustration, anger, or depression. The addition of a child places additional responsibilities of caregiving on both parents. Striking a balance between roles as a parent and worker, as well as resolving identity issues regarding these roles, is a process that can extend over years.

Throughout early to middle adulthood, parents focus on caring for and providing direction for their children. Parenting is difficult work; many adults are unprepared for the tasks of guiding and disciplining children toward success in personal relationships, school, or leisure activities. Most children successfully progress through childhood to their own adulthood, with only minor challenges for their parents along the way. Other children, however, struggle with learning or relationships throughout their childhood and their parents may be emotionally and cognitively challenged to change the course of events.

Throughout adulthood, partner relationships may be strained by events occurring with work, children, other family members, or friends. Just as their children are about to attain their independence, parents may find that their own aging parents need more help with independent living. Taking care of two generations is often a challenge of middle adulthood. The terms "sandwich generation" or "squeeze generation" are used to describe the situation in which one's children still retain the need for some guidance and assistance while one's parents are beginning to need more. This situation has occurred as a result of longer life spans of elders, delayed onset of childbearing, and longer periods of parenting responsibilities.

Throughout adulthood variables that influence health and well-being revolve around a person's physical abilities, economic or work responsibilities, and relationships with family, friends, and co-workers. The ability to find satisfaction in adult roles is often related to physical, social, emotional, and cognitive aspects of occupations familiar to an occupational therapy practitioner. Many opportunities exist to work with adults in the community in the areas of work, rehabilitation, and well-being. The types of community practice described here barely scratch the surface of possibilities for occupational therapy practitioners to enhance quality of life for individuals and populations in our communities.

COMMUNITY PRACTICES FOR ADULTS

We will describe four main foci of occupational therapy practitioners providing community service to adults:

- Ergonomics
- Return to work programs or welfare-to-work programs
- Home based rehabilitation
- Wellness programs

Ergonomics

Ergonomics takes an occupational therapy practitioner into the workplace to evaluate work procedures and design modifications that will help prevent injuries and enhance the productivity of workers. Most developed countries are engaged in growing their economies through increased productivity and developing new technologies. If these changes in work processes can be accomplished in a way that also reduces potential for injury and yields more productive workers, employers would be delighted. Occupational therapy practitioners working in the area of ergonomics use specialized skills and knowledge along with clinical reasoning to solve problems of work safety and productivity. They examine and analyze client and environmental factors as well as components of work related to performance and productivity. An example of this kind of occupational therapy practice is serving as a consultant to community businesses and organizations by identifying and providing interventions for repetitive motion injuries such as carpal tunnel syndrome, tendonitis, and back injury.

To be effective in this area of practice, a therapist must acquire some additional skills and knowledge. Although a business degree is not required, acquiring basic business knowledge and skills in marketing, economics, production, and management will ease the occupational therapy practitioner's transition to ergonomics or other emerging practice areas (Brachtesende, 2005). Understanding the economic impact of disease or injury and being able to communicate this to employers effectively is essential. Being able to explain how occupational therapy as either a direct or consultative service will save or generate money for an employer is another essential skill for those working in this area of practice. Effective communication and being able to speak the language of business makes this possible.

In 2002, the U.S. Department of Labor established guidelines for employers to improve ergonomics in the workplace. Although these guidelines are voluntary, there are advantages—including cost savings—for employers who consider implementing better work design and injury prevention programs (Brachtesende, 2005). To ease transition and ensure better fit into a workplace environment, an occupational therapy practitioner should understand the culture of the particular workplace. Community practice may require attention to such things as appropriate work attire. An occupational therapy practitioner dressing for work may wear work boots and a hard hat in one environment, and a business suit and briefcase in another. Being accepted in community practice often hinges on looking like you belong in the community rather than in a hospital.

Ergonomics is not an area of practice usually paid for with health care dollars. It is paid for by employers who see it as an adjustment that can save them money later on. In the current environment of sharing the costs of health care, injury prevention reduces the cost of health insurance premiums for the employer and employees. Since providing health care is one of the greatest costs associated with doing business in the United States, there is an incentive for businesses to put ergonomic or injury prevention programs in place. In addition to savings in healthcare costs, a worker who does not become injured can continue to perform his job. His employer will not need to compensate him for his injury nor will the employer have to hire and train another worker to do the job. Joss (2007) describes matching a person's functional abilities to job demands. This provides another opportunity for occupational therapy practitioners to work in the community providing ergonomics as a cost effective service to employers.

Occupational therapy practitioners bring a unique perspective to ergonomics. In addition to technical knowledge and skills of performance and person-environment fit, occupational therapy has at its roots the theory that a balance of work and rest are necessary to maintain maximal function (Nurit & Michal, 2003). Tucker, Folkard, and Macdonald (2003) stated that ergonomics practice emphasizing short rest breaks improves overall work performance, increases a worker's sense of well-being, and decreases accidents. Gravina, Lindstrom-Hazel, and Austin (2007) showed that ergonomic intervention resulted in improved worker safety.

An occupational therapy practitioner who chooses community practice in the area of ergonomics should be confident of her ability to communicate with business managers and workers, to enjoy problem solving, and to work both independently and collaboratively with non-healthcare workers. Challenges in the emerging community practice area of ergonomics include using occupations and evidence-based practice in evaluation and intervention, as well as demonstrating program effectiveness to employers and introducing them to the benefits of occupational therapy for their workers (Gerg & Smith, 2008).

Return to Work Programs

Work is a major focus of adult life. In adult socializing one of the first questions following introductions is "What do you do"? The type of work one does can be important when making new acquaintances because it seems to convey status in the community. Some people see work as a means to an end, such as when a person says, "I need a new job that allows me to also spend more time with my family," or "I need a job that pays more so that I can buy a new car," or "I need a job to support my family." Work in many ways defines the formal boundaries of adulthood. Adulthood begins with independence made possible by a first full-time job. The self-identity associated with work often ends with retirement from a job. Because work is so closely tied to self-identity and what we are able to do in our lives, it is a primary concern of many people who experience illness or disability and are temporarily unable to return to work. Work and employment is one of the major life areas defined in the *International Classification of Functioning, Disability and Health* (WHO, 2001).

Returning people to work reflects the early practice of occupational therapy, which included vocational rehabilitation to return people to a job following illness or injury. This area of occupational therapy practice continues to focus on either returning a person to work following a disabling injury or illness, or helping a person without a disability return to work or find a new job after a period of unemployment. As the world economy declines, more workers are finding themselves unemployed for longer periods of time, often accompanied by either determination to find future employment or despair that they may be unable to be as well-employed as in the past. Occupational therapy practitioners might consider how they can participate in addressing work issues such as re-training people for new work or addressing psychological barriers to future employment for workers whose jobs have ceased to exist.

Sager and James (2005) describe occupational therapy practitioners as having skills, knowledge, and philosophical base to maximize the best fit between a worker, a job, and an environment. This Australian study found that injured workers lacked knowledge and understanding about their injury and their rehabilitation process. They did not feel supported in their efforts to return to work because of dissatisfying task assignments and negative attitudes from peers and managers. Injured workers wanted to return to meaningful, productive work roles, and the authors suggested that occupational therapy practitioners had a responsibility to advocate for workers' successful return to work (Sager & James, 2005).

Return to work following a physical injury or illness is a goal of most adults. Personal identity and the ability to achieve and maintain financial independence are the main motivators for this goal. As with ergonomic practice, an employer's motivation for putting a disabled worker back to work is economic. Nighswonger (2000) reports that cost-benefit analysis reveals that rehabilitating and returning injured workers to work minimizes an employer's costs, even if workers are unable to do their previous jobs, or to do them as rapidly or effectively as they did prior to injury.

About 30 years ago, programs developed by physical and occupational therapists to return disabled workers to previous employment were called "work-hardening" programs. Initially offered in clinics or locations removed from the actual work environment, they focused on returning the worker to his job by incorporating injury prevention techniques into a program that gradually built the strength, endurance, range of motion, and dexterity necessary to perform the job. These early programs focused on a biomechanical model of practice while giving scant or no consideration to motivation and cognitive models of practice (Braverman, Sen & Kielhofner, 2001).

Although work-hardening programs reduced the effects of injury and built strength and endurance in workers who were required by their employers to attend these programs, workers remained unmotivated to return to their actual jobs. Loisel et al. (2005) assert that it is time to move worker rehabilitation away from a biomedical model focused on medical condition to a broader paradigm that accounts for the complexity of returning a person to work. Collaboration among therapy providers, coworkers, and managers to return a worker to the job site must begin as soon as possible after injury. This team should provide the worker with reassurance and grade intervention to control pain, while at the same time engaging the worker in meaningful and productive work in context (Loisel et al., 2005).

Rehabilitation that occurs at a worker's place of employment has the additional benefit of focusing attention on the prevention of further injuries to the worker and coworkers. Lysaght (2004) states that collaboration between therapists and insurance providers in a more global approach to return to work results in cost savings for both the employer and the insurance company. Lydell, Baigi, Marklund, and Mansson (2005) propose that reha- bilitation occurring shortly after injury, and involving skilled intervention in a timely manner, has a positive correlation with the worker's motivation to return to work and his success as a worker.

A holistic approach to returning workers to employment yields emotional benefits to the worker. When rehabilitation takes place in the employment environment, a worker can maintain connection to social aspects of work and his role as an employee at a familiar location. Many times work rela- tionships extend into leisure activities that can contribute to life satisfaction. When Johansson (2006) discusses the meaning of work for persons who have experienced a traumatic brain injury, a positive relationship with co- workers is cited as motivation for returning to work. After injury or illness, workers experience some anxiety about returning to their jobs, as the work itself may have been the cause of injury. The social dimensions of work, however, decrease anxiety associated with return to work and increase mean- ing of work and leisure activities.

When return to work happens soon after injury, work habits such as at- tendance and adhering to work rules are not disrupted. If the worker has the habit of stopping on the way home at the end of the work day to have a beer with his coworkers, this habit may continue. The worker also continues to receive pay for his work and is not given the opportunity to adapt to re- ceiving compensation from his employer for recovering at home. In work- hardening programs, which were clinically-based medical model practices, many workers stated that they received sufficient pay even when not work- ing and they didn't have to get up in the morning to do a job. Therefore they saw no reason to "get well" and go back to work.

Work can be regarded as a means to rehabilitation and also as an incen- tive to return to one's former patterns of work life. For most adults, work lends temporal and social structure to life and it gives one value and worth both monetarily and nonmonetarily.

Welfare-to-Work Programs

In the United States, a 1996 federal mandate requires persons receiving wel- fare to find a job. This program was called the Temporary Assistance to Needy Families (TANF) and its purpose was to replace government assis- tance with earned wages for about two million families (Rice & Wicks, 2006). The intent was to decrease the government burden of providing economic sustenance for those who were able to work but chose not to work. If a wel- fare recipient could not find a job or did not actively seek a job, he would lose his government benefits. Although logical in intent, the realities of this program adversely affected poor women and children as well as those with poor health, substandard education, mental illness, and substance abuse (Blocker & Freudenberg, 2001). TANF forced unemployed welfare recipients into the workplace. Once employed, however, they were often unable to keep their jobs as they lacked the ability to perform required tasks. The primary reasons for losing jobs had more to do with work habits than with specific job skills; many of the jobs these people found were low-skilled jobs. In addition, many unemployed persons had chronic problems in obtaining and keeping a job because of disabilities, domestic violence, and lack of family or other community support for their role as worker. For many welfare recipients, finding affordable child care was an insurmountable task and there is evidence that welfare-to-work experiences have had a negative impact on children of mothers required to work under this plan (Neblett, 2007).

The culture of poverty and unemployment remains the main disincentive to work; generations of families have lived on welfare and learned to rely on others to support them. New strategies to break this cycle are needed (Mallon, 2007). Providing motivation for unemployed persons to seek and maintain jobs is the challenge of many community workers. Although few occupational therapy practitioners participate in welfare-to-work programs, they can design and implement programs that address challenges of chronic unemployment, while utilizing a client-centered model to understand client needs and empower them to address performance problems.

Case management of clients who have been affected by TANF has had varied success. Hasenfeld (2004) stated that intensive case management centered on the client-case manager relationship was needed to get chronically unemployed persons into steady work. However, Jagannathan and Camasso (2006) found that public assistance workers assigned to help people transition from welfare to work lacked confidence in their own abilities. This was attributed to dissatisfaction with their organization's methods of expenditure, as well as to the disrespect public assistance workers felt they received from their clients and others involved in welfare-to-work programs. In order to achieve greater success rates, it was proposed that public assistance workers needed to expect their efforts to lead to success, which would in turn be recognized and rewarded by their employers (Jagannathan & Camasso, 2006).

Occupational therapy practitioners have worked as job coaches for persons with developmental disabilities. Similarities appear in programs designed for disabled persons and those designed for persons who have been chronically unemployed. Hasenfeld (2004) says that effectiveness in welfare-to-work programs requires one to be able to tailor a job to a client's particular needs.

One also needs the capacity to access and mobilize client and community internal and external resources, and the skills and knowledge to develop innovative service models.

When transitioning developmentally disabled clients into a job, an occupational therapy practitioner acting as a job coach will learn the demands of the job and make success more likely by using activity analysis to fit the job to the client. The therapist may not change the worker; rather she may change the job to fit the worker's abilities. Teaching work skills and including activities of daily living and instrumental activities of daily living, such as time management and social skills, are also part of the coach's job (Siporin & Lysack, 2004). Some preparation for work may occur in a classroom environment but most intervention occurs on the job and in the community. A job coach may teach a skill and model it for the worker, then assist the worker to do the job, using verbal or visual cues, until the job is performed adequately to lead to independent work. From time to time, however, as new tasks are added to the job or circumstances in a worker's life lead to unsatisfactory job performance, the coach may return briefly to get the worker back to an adequate level of job performance. Occupational therapy practitioners who serve as job coaches also need to work with client family members and others in the community to help them understand the benefits of engaging clients in work in the community (Siporin & Lysack, 2004).

The skills and knowledge of a job coach are similar to those required to get persons on welfare into the workplace. Blitz and Mechanic (2006) say job coaches are hired by community agencies to provide specialized job training and ongoing support for the client to learn, perform, and adjust to the work environment. Job coaches need skills and knowledge to develop business and community connections that can help provide employment and support clients in the community. They also need sufficient skills and knowledge to facilitate decision-making in clients, teach skills, and continue to monitor and respond to changes in the client or the work environment over time (Blitz & Mechanic, 2006; Howarth, Mann, Huafeng, McDermott & Butkus, 2006).

Some of the specific requirements for individuals who are transitioning from welfare to work include activities of daily living, such as hygiene and grooming appropriate for the workplace. Social and communication skills may need to be developed to assist a client to adapt to a work culture. Training in work routines, especially time management, is very important to maintaining a job. In order to keep a job, one must show up to work at the scheduled time, adhere to scheduled breaks, and work a specific number of hours. If one has never held a job, these may be new concepts. There may never have been consequences for not showing up or being late for an appointment.

Learning workplace socialization is another habit that may need to be taught. A person may need to learn to greet and thank others and be polite even if they feel disinclined to do so. An occupational therapy practitioner can match a person's skills and abilities to specific demands of a particular job by using an occupational profile and observations of the work environment. Once a person begins to experience success in work performance, establishes meaningful relationships with coworkers, and collects a paycheck, that person begins to change his perception of worth and value to society. Success is a great motivator for people; personal causation makes changes possible and continues to support change (Kielhofner, 2002).

Facilitating people to become engaged in meaningful work is an appropriate role for occupational therapy practitioners who want to work in the community. Seeing and acting on the possibilities for changing the lives of people through occupation is rewarding work, but requires flexibility and patience with persons who may appear unmotivated to work. The ability to modify work environments to assure successful performance includes gathering specialized knowledge about the work itself and determining how the use of technology might enhance performance. Return-to-work programs are rarely covered under private healthcare plans, but instead receive funding from employers, local and national government programs, or community initiatives. The potential for work in this area is determined by community economic climate. In a tight job market, for example, fewer jobs may be available to persons with challenging work patterns, and agencies may have fewer resources to compensate job coaches (Howarth, Mann, Huafeng, McDermott & Butkus, 2006).

HOME HEALTH REHABILITATION

Adults injured in an accident or disabled as a result of illness or acute medical condition may be sent to a rehabilitation or similar facility soon after stabilization in a hospital. Some persons, however, may want to return home for rehabilitation. In order to qualify for private health insurance funding, home health services generally follow a medical model of treatment. Most agencies that offer home care services employ nurses to facilitate a patient's recovery, and also include the rehabilitation services of occupational, physical, and speech therapists. Visits occur in the client's home and may be scheduled for one or more times a week, depending upon how much funding is allocated based on a client's need for services.

The principles of evaluation and intervention in home health rehabilitation are the same principles used in hospital settings. The instruments used for evaluation are the same. The context of treatment, however, may differ. When working in a client's home, the service provider is not in control of the experience; she does not have clinic equipment to use and cannot control the environment's temperature, noise, light level, or cleanliness. The client, or the client's family, controls their home environment, goals for intervention, and to some extent, the intervention methods. Appointment times may be determined by the client and his family. The occupational therapy practitioner is invited into the client's environment, and is treated as both a guest and employee of the client and his family (Gifford, Wooster, Gray & Chromiak, 2001). While differences exist between hospital and home rehabilitation, Mitchell and Unsworth (2004) remind occupational therapy practitioners that community service requires the same accountability as institutional care. This includes accountability for evaluation, intervention, and documentation. Sources of payment and reimbursement for home health services require that these tasks remain the same no matter where the service is provided.

When providing therapy within a home environment, a client may be allowed to perform tasks in a preferred location. If cooking is a priority for the client, this can be carried out in his home kitchen. Doing so may require relocation of cooking equipment, reorganization of appliances, or modification of cooking techniques to accommodate disability, but the client collaborates in these decisions. Seeing the kitchen's actual condition helps the therapist make more effective recommendations than would be possible otherwise. Performance skills, context, and environment related to performance of these occupations can also be addressed more effectively when the client's home facilities are used during intervention. Problems that arise in performance may be addressed and modifications made to facilitate maximum independence in a natural environment.

Client motivation to perform may also be different at home than in the hospital. An adult rehabilitation client may have family members living with her who can help her continue in roles that are important to her and her family. If a mother becomes disabled and can no longer perform certain instrumental activities of daily living such as housecleaning or laundry, she can instruct others how to perform these tasks and can be available to listen and give advice. Isolation and loss of a valued role, on the other hand, can lead to loss of identity, depression, and associated problems. Client's performance supports personal needs and a valued role.

UNIVERSAL DESIGN IN HOMES AND PUBLIC SPACES

One advantage to rehabilitating a client in his home is the opportunity to observe barriers that constrain functional performance. Barriers that the client must live with become evident to the therapist—even barriers the client or family members may not be aware can be removed. If the client uses a wheelchair, for example, it may not fit through doorways into the home, or from one room to another. The bathroom or kitchen may not be accessible.

Occupational therapy practitioners who introduce clients and their families to universal design can make home life easier for everyone. Universal design means the creation and use of environments and products that make homes and communities accessible for all people. High costs of specialized products made for persons with disabilities, coupled with an aging population of adults who want to make their home environments accommodate any future decline in performance ability, led to the development and marketing of a broad range of commercial products that could be produced and sold for less (The Center for Universal Design, 2008). Universal design has been embraced by persons of all ages with and without disabilities, including parents of children with special needs who want to make their home equally accessible to their entire family.

Liao (2008) describes a kitchen remodeling that used universal design to accommodate family members of significantly differing heights. The family wanted a kitchen that was attractive, functional, and designed not to decrease resale value of their home. The home owner sought a person knowledgeable about universal design to redesign her kitchen and coordinate with contractors and manufacturers of kitchen furnishings.

A Story from Practice

I arrived at the home of a client with multiple sclerosis and saw that her front door was at street level. "Great," I thought, "She lives on the ground floor and does not have to worry about stairs." Located right inside the front door was the bathroom. Immediately after, however, I encountered two steps down to her main living area, which included her bedroom and kitchen. To use the bathroom, my client had to negotiate two steps, and this had begun to be a challenge. Railings were installed next to the steps to keep her from falling, but when she began to use a wheelchair, it became clear that this housing arrangement made her bathroom and toilet inaccessible to her. She could not get up the stairs with the wheelchair, and even with a ramp the doorways were too narrow and the room too small to accommodate a wheelchair. The temporary use of a bedside commode in the client's bedroom met her toileting needs for the time being, but addressing this client's long-term toileting and bathing needs required finding more suitable housing that put her entire living area on one level with doors and rooms wide enough to accommodate wheelchair use.

Home modifications have long been an area of occupational therapy practice. In home health rehabilitation, the occupational therapy practitioner works with the family to make adjustments to their home to safely accommodate a client's needs. Many older adults are modifying their current homes, and new home construction often embraces principles of universal design. However, when builders approach design of a home to accommodate disabilities, they may not be thorough in their approach.

A Story from Practice

When I was looking at some new homes, I found that many featured walk-in showers without thresholds, flip handles on doors and bath and kitchen fixtures, and lowered electrical outlets. One home I visited included a separate living area for a live-in caretaker. The builder of this home discussed how ideal the home would be for an aging person who might have a disability. He pointed out all of the accessible features of the home, including an elevator installed to move a resident from one floor of the home to another. He should have consulted an occupational therapy practitioner. I pointed out to the builder that once inside the home the homeowner would be able to be independent, but the two entrances to the home each had four steps and there was no space to install any type of ramp. It's great to be able to be independent in one's own home, but not so good to be trapped inside it.

Occupational therapy practitioners may find opportunities to collaborate not only with individuals seeking universal design in their homes, but also with engineers and architects challenged by not understanding benefits of incorporating universal design into public places. Some architects believe that universal design may compromise the look they seek in their building (Skinner, 2008). By helping designers of public spaces to understand the effects of their plans on all people who may use the space, designs can be modified to improve the functionality of community spaces.

While helping create accessible living spaces and increasing access to public spaces for everyone, occupational therapy practitioners will work with a variety of people unfamiliar with the performance needs of persons with differing abilities. As they facilitate better understanding of space requirements of some universal design features, occupational therapy practitioners can assist builders to weigh the benefits of universal design against the costs of construction. Home projects that may seem simple to homeowners may be more complicated than envisioned, and if done incorrectly may not benefit the people who would use them (Felix, 2008). Working with home-owners, interior and building designers, and contractors to tackle projects incorporating universal design allows occupational therapy practitioners to bring benefits of access to everyone who uses private or public spaces in the community.

WELLNESS PROGRAMS

The World Health Organization defines well-being to include all aspects of a person's life, including physical, mental, and social abilities related to participation in life activities (WHO, 2001). The *International Classification of Functioning, Disability and Health* (ICF) provides a classification framework to understand and study health and related areas such as disability prevention and health promotion (WHO, 2001). Prevention of physical and mental disabilities through community intervention and wellness programs promotes health and well-being (Russell & Lloyd, 2004). Programs to promote wellness might include eliminating risk factors such as obesity through weight control and exercise programs, and working to reduce unhealthy levels of stress. Ideally these services will be offered in supportive community environments.

As some adults transition through the middle years of life, they become less physically active than in earlier stages. Work and family responsibilities may cause role strain where a person simply has too much to do and not enough time in which to do it. An overscheduled person may feel that she is not performing adequately and be quite dissatisfied with her role performance. Job insecurity in a changing economic environment may cause workers to work harder and harder in an attempt to retain job security. Many workers forego vacations or rest periods, thinking this practice will help preserve their jobs. They may spend less time engaged in leisure activities or with their families. They may not eat whole meals but rather snack on unhealthy food in their cars or at their desks because it takes less time and they can return to work more quickly. All of these lifestyle choices may contribute to the development of chronic diseases that may become disabling (Folland, Goodman & Stano, 2007).

The benefits of wellness extend from the individual to the community and to society. Obesity-related chronic health problems or acute illnesses—such as diabetes and cardiovascular disease—result in death for some, but for many more people result in a remaining lifetime with disability. A person may lose a job he is no longer able to perform, be unable to participate in family or community activities, and may experience depression. The cost of caring for a person with a chronic disabling condition is significant, and is one that many communities are no longer able to absorb. Occupational therapy practitioners therefore may make a significant social and economic impact on their communities by offering wellness programs sponsored by agencies or employers who want to improve the health and well-being of their constituents.

Occupational therapy practitioners have begun to offer more community services intended to minimize the effects of lifestyle illnesses. As they consider the long-term needs of populations and contribute to building healthier communities, occupational therapy practitioners will need to work collaboratively with other professionals in developing health policy directed toward wellness (Baum & Law, 1998). Wellness programs vary widely, but most occupational therapy practitioners stress the importance of maintaining balance in work, self-care, and leisure activities to give meaning to life and to sustain productivity. Occupational therapy practitioner can advocate for access to community programs that facilitate wellness for persons with and without disabilities. In such programs, they would act as consultants rather than primary practitioners (Russell & Lloyd, 2004).

Neufeld and Kneipman (2001) describe a community program they collaboratively developed with an organization serving persons with a diagnosis of multiple sclerosis. The purpose of the program was to establish patterns of wellness for adults with chronic disabling conditions. Designed in collaboration with clients, the program empowered clients through participatory learning and active involvement as both providers and consumers of services. Participants learned about their illness, established personal goals, and participated in an exercise program to maintain physical endurance and flexibility. They learned the importance of balance in life activities, how to adapt their home environments to simplify tasks, how to maintain valued roles, and how to cope with the symptoms of their illness.

Another wellness program developed by an occupational therapy practitioner stressed her strong belief in each individual's need to assume personal responsibility for his or her own wellness. This program, based on the therapist's professional experiences and her personal participation in wellness activities, was offered through an existing community agency. The program was geared toward active participation rather than classroom lectures, and included activities focused on nutrition, exercise, and stress reduction. Enjoying and fully participating in activities was an important part of the program. The occupational therapist who developed it intends to become self employed providing wellness programs to people in her community.

Russell and Lloyd (2004) describe a program developed to promote wellness in persons diagnosed with mental illness. Offered through an existing continuing education program in the community, it was designed to improve access and promote inclusion of persons with mental illness in free or low-cost educational, recreational, and vocational services. Occupational therapy practitioners worked collaboratively with participants to identify goals including weight loss, fitness, and acquisition of job skills. Courses were developed to enhance self-esteem, establish personal goals, manage time, reduce stress, and improve motivation, life skills, nutrition, and relaxation. This program succeeded in engaging persons with mental illness toward meeting their personal goals and furthered their community engagement through participation in other educational and recreational activities. The program helped return some participants to employment.

Occupational therapy practitioners are offering yoga, tai chi, or similar physical activities through community agencies or fitness centers. These activities promote balance, strength, and a sense of well-being, and are designed to include persons with disabilities. Helping people to understand the importance of balance in their lives and to include time for renewal, relaxation, and physical activity is an important component of occupational therapy. Persons of varying ages, from childhood through old age, can participate in these activities. Adults of any age, therefore, have the opportunity to avoid or minimize chronic health problems by changing their patterns of living.

LIFE COACHING

Life coaching is a developing specialty within occupational therapy community practice. This service helps clients achieve wellness in a challenging environment. Work-related stress is known to affect personal performance adversely. Life coaching can mediate stress to the benefit of clients and their employers (Hawksley, 2007). Coaches assist their clients to find better balance in personal and professional life, to clarify short and longer term personal and professional goals, solve problems, increase energy, and stay focused on achieving greater satisfaction with life (Yousey, 2001). A life coach may facilitate a client to identify and plan steps to achieve a goal that may seem elusive without structured assistance. The coaching process is one of collaboration and trust in which the coach uses her skills to help identify challenges, propose solutions, and facilitate the client in problem solving. Empowering the client to achieve his goals and enhance life satisfaction is the role of the coach (Yousey, 2001).

What skills, knowledge, and personal characteristics does an occupational therapy practitioner wanting to offer wellness programs in the community need? She must be knowledgeable about lifestyle diseases as well as environmental challenges and supports, and have the collaborative skills to work with others outside the healthcare environment. She may also choose to offer her own personal experiences with wellness practices and skills as examples to her clients to enhance their own wellness. Most people who become providers in this area of practice serve as role models for their clients. They manage their own health first through achieving balance in life, engaging in healthy eating, and participating in regular exercise and relaxation. Working with persons engaged in changing their ways of living requires a therapist who can facilitate the client's personal motivation. If a person slips back into unhealthy patterns of living, a therapist must be nonjudgmental and continue to encourage possibilities for change. Involvement in wellness programs requires a therapist with good collaboration skills who can work with agencies and employers seeking these services for clients or employees.

CHAPTER SUMMARY

Working with adults either in long established or innovative community programs provides an opportunity for occupational therapy practitioners to utilize old and new skills and knowledge, and collaborate with clients and community agencies. Most community practice therapists find their work especially rewarding. It allows a long-term relationship with clients, offers challenging opportunities to solve problems with clients, and allows various degrees of work autonomy and diversity each day. Although this chapter provides a few examples of the types of work available in community practice, many other opportunities exist to enhance quality of life for adults in our communities.

LEARNING ACTIVITIES

Adulthood spans many years and is a mosaic of tasks and challenges that are not necessarily sequential. Social and economic factors have become highly unpredictable, and can alter progression of personal plans. Community practice opportunities arise from the tasks of adulthood and the challenges that alter a person's plans. Identifying these challenges may lead to ideas for community practice to benefit individuals and groups.

1. A challenge for workers in an economy that is declining after years of prosperity is loss of jobs. Identify the physical, social, and psychological effects of job loss for:

   - A man or woman who is the sole financial provider for a family
   - A man or woman whose primary role is to care for home and family
   - A recent college graduate who is unable to find employment
   - A man or woman who is about 50 years old, has no dependents, but has planned for early retirement

2. Lifestyle choices can lead to health concerns that increase healthcare costs and lower life expectancy. These are concerns for an entire community to address. Identify specific lifestyle choices that are problematic in your community and suggest wellness programs to address these concerns for individuals and community.
3. Explore your community and identify available programs to improve wellness. What specific services or activities are offered? How might an occupational therapy practitioner enhance these services?
4. An adult may be engaged in parenting a dependent child and at the same time be caring for aging parents. Describe how the responsibility of caring for two generations may produce stress for the caregiver. What would community practice designed for this caregiver look like? How might this type of practice be structured to financially support a service provider?
5. The economic decline has been accompanied by high unemployment. Occupational therapy practitioners may develop services to assist those who are recently unemployed or workers who have had prolonged periods of unemployment. What are some of the services or interventions that might be offered to unemployed persons? Design an outcome study to show the efficacy of these interventions to address the problem of high unemployment.

REFERENCES

Baum, C. & Law, M. (1998). Nationally speaking: Community health: A responsibility, an opportunity and a fit for occupational therapy. *American Journal of Occupational Therapy, 52* (1) 7–10.

Blitz, C.L. & Mechanic, D. (2006). Facilitators and barriers to employment among individuals with psychiatric disabilities: A job coach perspective. *Work, 26* (4) 407–419.

Blocker, D.E. & Freudenberg, N. (2001). Developing comprehensive approaches to prevention and control of obesity among low-income, urban, African-American women. *Journal of the American Medical Women's Association, 56* (2) 59–64.

Brachtesende, A. (2005). New markets emerge from society's needs. *OT Practice, 10* (1) 17–18.

Braverman, B.H., Sen, S.S. & Kielhofner, G. (2001). Community based work programs. In M. Scaffa (Ed.) *Occupational therapy in community-based settings.* pp. 139–162. Philadelphia, PA: F.A. Davis.

Felix, L. (2008). Design for everyone. *Library Journal, 133* (16) 38–40.

Folland. S., Goodman, A.C. & Stano, M. (2007). *The economics of health and health care (5th ed).* Upper Saddle River, NJ: Prentice Hall.

Gerg, M.J. & Smith, S. (2008). Training the "industrial athlete": Developing job-specific exercise programs to reduce injuries. *OT Practice, 13* (7) CE1–CE8.

Gifford, K.E., Wooster, D.A, Gray, L. & Chromiak, S.B. (2001). Home health. In M. Scaffa (Ed.) *Occupational therapy in community based settings.* pp. 188–222. Philadelphia, PA: F.A. Davis.

Gravina, N., Lindstrom-Hazel, D. & Austin, J. (2007). The effects of workstation changes and behavioral interventions on safe typing postures in an office. *Work, 29* (3) 245–253.

Hasenfeld, Y. & Evans Powell, L. (2004). The role of non-profit agencies in the provision of welfare-to-work services. *Administration in Social Work, 4* (3) 309–326.

Hawksley, B. (2007). Work-related stress, work/life balance and personal life coaching. *British Journal of Nursing, 12* (1) 34–36.

Howarth, E., Mann, J.R., Huafeng, Z, McDermott, S. & Butkus, S. (2006). What predicts re-employment after job loss for individuals with mental retardation? *Journal of Vocational Rehabilitation, 24* (3) 183–189.

Jagannathan, R. & Camasso, M. (2006). Public assistance workers' confidence in welfare-to-work programs and the clients they serve. *Administration in Social Work, 30* (1) 7–32.

Johansson, U. & Tham, K. (2006). The meaning of work after acquired brain injury. *American Journal of Occupational Therapy, 60* (1) 60–69.

Joss, M. (2007). The importance of job analysis in occupational therapy. *British Journal of Occupational Therapy, 70* (7) 301–303.

Kielhofner, G. (2002). *A model of human occupation: Theory and application.* Baltimore, MD: Lippincott, Williams & Wilkins.

Liao, A. (2008). Heightened awareness. *Kitchen and Bath Business, 55* (9) 68–69.

Loisel, P., Falardeau, M., Baril, R., Jose-Durnad, M., Langley, A., Sauve, S. & Gervais, J. (2005). The values underlying team decision-making in work rehabilitation for musculoskeletal disorders. *Disability and Rehabilitation, 37* (10) 561–569.

Lydell, M., Baigi, A., Markland, B. & Mansson, J. (2005). Predictive factors for work capacity in patients with musculoskeletal disorders. *Journal of Rehabilitation Medicine, 23* (2) 139–146.

Lysaght, R. (2004). Approaches to worker rehabilitation by occupational and physical therapists in the United Sates: Factors impacting practice. *Work, 23* (2) 139–146.

Mallon, A.J. (2007). Employers and work first policies: Exploring workplace support practices. *Journal of Policy Practice, 6* (4) 3–24.

Mitchell, R. & Unsworth, C.A. (2004). Role perceptions and clinical reasoning of community health occupational therapists undertaking home visits. *Australian Occupational Therapy Journal, 51* (1) 13–24.

Neblett, N.G. (2007). Patterns of single mothers' work and welfare use. What matters most for children's well-being? *Journal of Family Issues, 28* (8) 1083–1112.

Neufeld, P. & Kneipman, K. (2001). Gateway to wellness: An occupational therapy collaboration with the National Multiple Sclerosis Society. *Occupational Therapy in Health Care, 13* (3/4) 67–84.

Nighswonger, T. (2000). Research shows fast return to work is best. *Occupational Hazards, 62,* 26–28.

Nurit, W. & Michal, A-R. (2003). Rest: A qualitative exploration of the phenomenon. *Occupational Therapy International, 10* (4) 227–238.

Peters, T. (2005). *Re-imagine! Business excellence in a disruptive age.* London: Dorling Kindersley, Limited.

Rice, M. & Wicks, M. (2006). Assessing the health of women moving from welfare to work. *AWHONN Lifelines, 9* (6) 468–472.

Russell, A. & Lloyd, C. (2004). Partnerships in mental health: Addressing barriers to social inclusion. *International Journal of Therapy and Rehabilitation, 11* (6) 267–274.

Sager, L. & James, C. (2005). Injured workers' perspectives of their rehabilitation process under the New South Wales workers compensation system. *Australian Occupational Therapy Journal, 52* (2) 127–135.

Skinner, J. (2008). Public places, universal spaces. *Planning 74* (7) 10–13.

Siporin, S. & Lysack, C. (2004). Quality of life and supported employment: A case study of three women with developmental disabilities. *The American Journal of Occupational Therapy, 58* (4) 455–465.

The Center for Universal Design (2008). The history of universal design. Raleigh, NC: The Center for Universal Design. Retrieved October 31, 2008 from http://www.design.ncsu.edu/cud_about_ud/uhistory.html.

Tucker, P., Folkard, S. & Macdonald, I. (2003). Rest breaks and accident risk. *Lancet, 361* (9358) 680.

World Health Organization (2001). *International classification of functioning, disability and health.* Geneva, Switzerland: World Health Organization.

Yousey, J. (2001). Life coaching: A one to one approach to changing lives. *OT Practice, 6* (1) 11–14.

Chapter 5

Aging in the Community

- Associate aging-related changes with opportunities to provide community services.
- Explore existing community practices with aging adults.
- Demonstrate that people with differing abilities have different priorities for services as they age.

INTRODUCTION

Adulthood, a period of industry and life changes, evolves through the process of aging. At no specific point in time does one say "I am old." Aging is a gradual process subject to health and well-being. Newspapers and news shows abound with stories about the approaching costs to society associated with aging "baby-boomers," Yet many of these "boomers" do not see themselves as old, nor do they anticipate significant changes occurring in their lifestyles. Of the approximately 78 million baby boomers, pre-seniors, or those ages 55 to 64, are expected to increase 50% between 2000 and 2010 (Bouk, 2008). Many older people continue to age without any disability or significant changes in their occupations. They continue to care for themselves, to work at paid or volunteer jobs, and to engage in leisure activities with a variety of people of all ages. Statistics associated with aging, however, reveal that about one-half of the older population will develop at least one disability. As people continue to live longer, we can anticipate an increased incidence of disability in the oldest people in our communities (Bass-Haugen, Henderson, Larson & Matuska, 2005). Freedman, Martin, Schoeni, and Cornman (2008), however, more encouragingly report that fewer people 75 years of age and older report difficulty with activities of daily living.

DEVELOPMENTAL ROLES AND CHALLENGES OF AGING

It is difficult to classify people who are aging as old, or the elderly as belonging to a specific age group. One is eligible to be a member of the American Association of Retired Persons (AARP) at age 50 and receive special discounts at stores or entertainment venues at age 63 or 65. The government has gradually been increasing the age of retirement, with most baby boomers eligible to retire at age 67. Yet these same people must register for Medicare at age 65, and most businesses do not have a mandatory retirement age. People over 70 years of age continue to be engaged as leaders in business, the arts, and government. Aging, therefore, may be an individual construct rather than one defined by society.

Physical Changes of Aging

Adults experience physical changes associated with aging, including diminished sensations of vision, hearing, smell, and taste. They may experience joint damage due to obesity or hard use over time. As they age, many people must cope with arthritis and its associated pain and joint immobility. Even as this process occurs, most aging adults continue to engage in lifelong activities such as keyboarding, needlework, or running until these activities become so painful that they are no longer enjoyed. In some cases, pain relievers and joint replacement enable people to return to their former occupations with pain and deformity relieved. The incidence of cardiovascular disease, heart attack, and stroke also increases with age. The disability and physical limitations that sometimes accompany these conditions may be overcome with rehabilitation. In some cases, however, lives are changed dramatically by cardiovascular incidents that render aging adults no longer able to care for themselves. Significant changes in living arrangements may result.

People with chronic illnesses such as Parkinson's disease or multiple sclerosis experience increasing disability with age and begin to require more care. The aging process can also alter cognition. Aging adults may begin gradually exhibiting symptoms of dementia or Alzheimer's disease. An estimated 5 million, or one in eight, baby boomers will develop Alzheimer's disease (Salloway,

Feldman, Kandian & De Kosky, 2008; Cajigal, 2008). The risk of developing Alzheimer's dementia increases with age, doubling for each five-year span after age 65 until nearly half of individuals older than age 85 have the disease (Bren, 2003). Plassman et al. (2008) report that 22.2% of all persons over age 71 had cognitive impairment without dementia, which is associated with increased risk of disability, increased healthcare costs, and progression to dementia.

Economics of Aging

One major life transition that has for many years characterized aging is retirement from paid employment. Retirement is welcomed by some and is approached anxiously by those who have failed to prepare for it. One factor that influences how retirement is experienced is the financial status of an aging adult. When a person has the financial means not to worry about his future, retirement may be a time to engage in activities such as travel or hobbies that were impossible during the years of paid employment. Many retirement communities are built around active participation in a variety of activities intended for adults in their late fifties and older who have the means to move into these communities. Financial security, however, does not guarantee a successful retirement. If a person has not developed meaningful hobbies, sports, or other interests outside of work, retirement can be a difficult period. A person who identifies himself with his job, or who has spent his entire adult life engaged in a career, may find that after retirement he has nothing to fill the empty hours that had been occupied by paid employment.

Many aging adults face financial difficulties at the time of retirement. They may not have a pension plan, a pension they expected is no longer available, or they have not saved money for retirement. It is difficult to live on social and employee benefits that were designed for a time when life expectancy was much shorter than it is today (Turner, 2008). Dependence on government programs results in many aging adults living near the poverty level. Many of these people, who would prefer to retire, must continue to work to survive and their work must be designed to accommodate their age-related needs. People who thought they would enjoy a financially stable retirement suddenly may find themselves without financial means to retire as companies file for bankruptcy and pension plans are scaled back or cut entirely. Additionally, public policy encourages aging adults to remain in the workplace longer and retire at an older age (Turner, 2008). Within a very short time, however, recent international economic trends have created large numbers of unemployed workers and high unemployment rates, which may make it more difficult for aging adults to remain in the workplace.

Changes in Life Roles

Life roles may also change with aging. If a wife develops Alzheimer's disease, her husband may need to care for her and their home. This is a role reversal of their previous living situation in which the wife was the caregiver and homemaker while the husband worked outside the home. As people live longer, some aging adults find themselves caring for even older parents. This may prove difficult for an adult child experiencing diminished physical abilities due to arthritis, high blood pressure, or other chronic conditions that can make physical care of an older parent painful and difficult. Fuhr, Martinez and Williams (2008) report that 44.4 million informal caregivers are responsible for family members with chronic health conditions, a service valued at more than $257 billion a year. Bull and McShane (2008) report that 80 percent of long-term care for elders is provided by family members. Life roles of parent and child also may be reversed as a child becomes the caregiver, a role traditionally ascribed to the parent. Giving care to an older parent or disabled spouse is stressful and may require the caregiver to give up some personally meaningful activities such as work, leisure activities, and socialization outside the home. All these activities contribute to a sense of well-being and promote health. (Gitlin, Corcoran, Winter, Boyce & Marcus, 1999).

Quality of Life

Quality of life remains as important throughout the aging process as it is in earlier stages of life. Lau and McKenna (2001) studied a group of elders living in Hong Kong who had each experienced a stroke. They compared their quality of life to elders who had survived a stroke and were living in other countries, as well as to elders who had not experienced a disabling condition. They found that for all elders a positive relationship exists between engagement in activity and subsequent mental health, and that this relationship contributes to quality of life. People who continue to live in their communities and remain active are more satisfied with their lives in general. Participation in instrumental activities of daily living and leisure were important to aging adults. Elders who had high prevalence of depression, anxiety, and irritability experienced decreased quality of life, while those who felt positive about themselves retained a sense of control, good coping mechanisms, and greater satisfaction with their lives. When cognitive dysfunction occurs as a result of disease or acute illness it results in decreased social function, diminished roles, increased depression, and a poorer quality of life. Haak, Fange, Horstmann and Iwarsson (2008) report that an independent home life, along with active engagement in community social activities, decreased depression and mortality in the very old. Timmons (2008) reports that programs engaging aging adults in physical and cognitive activities and socialization pay for themselves by increasing health and decreasing need for prescription drugs and hospital stays.

Socioeconomic status influences quality of life in aging adults. Lau and McKenna (2001) describe the adverse effect of poverty on Hong Kong elders who do not receive a pension or have family nearby to assist them. Socioeconomic status affected quality of life for aging adults in the United States more than for those in Canada (Huguet, Kaplan & Feeny, 2008). This was thought to result from differences in access to health care and greater socioeconomic inequality within the two countries. Worsening economic conditions would likely have an adverse effect on elders throughout the world, but would likely have a more profound effect in the United States due to disparities in health care and income. In the United States, the high cost of prescription medications has made living with a chronic condition more difficult for lower income elders. Even with assistance from government programs, some medications are beyond the means of low income elders, and many aging adults find government payment for health care difficult to understand. As a consequence of the financial difficulty of obtaining prescription medicines, some aging adults have resorted to skipping doses or breaking tablets in half in an attempt to make the medication they have available last longer. Either of these practices can lead to ill health and often necessitate more costly health care.

Spirituality has been found to contribute to quality of life for aging adults. Spirituality includes a personal belief system that may or may not be related to religion (Lau & McKenna, 2001). This finding from the study of Hong Kong elders has been further supported by other literature about the positive influence of spirituality and religious beliefs on life satisfaction in aging adults. Latin American and Caribbean elders reported religious affiliation to be very important in their lives. Reyes-Ortiz, Peleaz, Koenig and Mulligan, (2008) stated that people who were more religious reported themselves to have better health and had higher levels of function than those who were less religious. Wang, Chan, Ng, and Ho (2008) studied aging Chinese adults with vision impairments and found that spirituality had a positive effect on general physical and mental health, and aided the elders' adaptation to vision loss. Although attending to spiritual needs of clients of any age is important, it seems to be especially important to address with aging adults.

Engagement in leisure activities enhances quality of life throughout the life span, but a link has been established between successful aging and participation in serious leisure (Brown, McGuire & Voelkl, 2008). Serious leisure is defined as activity that requires a high level of active participation, provides an outlet for creativity, and offers opportunities for playfulness and lifelong learning (Vallant, 2002). The demands of serious leisure resemble the acquisition of skills and knowledge required to develop a career. An aging adult engaged in serious leisure would learn and be challenged to succeed. The result would be feelings of accomplishment and an identification as a practitioner of the leisure activity (Vallant, 2002).

Just as in earlier stages, aging adults must respond to changes in the environment that are beyond their control. Aging may include the loss of physical or cognitive abilities, of employment, or of financial security after retirement. Social participation may decrease as friends and family relocate or die. Throughout the aging process, elders continue to need engagement in meaningful and purposeful activities, even as these activities may become difficult due to illness or the need to provide care for a family member. As they age, most people want to continue to live at home, to participate in their communities, and to enjoy their lives.

SOME COMMUNITY PRACTICE OPTIONS

Many opportunities exist for occupational therapy practitioners in community practice to work with aging adults. Occupational therapy practitioners who have focused their careers on study and work with aging adults will know of services needed in the community that can lead to development of a community practice. Textbooks focused on aging and community services offered by occupational therapy practitioners will identify both individual and collective needs of aging adults and any related opportunities for community practice (Bonder, Dal Bello-Haas & Wagner, 2009). This chapter describes a few examples of occupational therapy practice in the community with aging adults; however, this discussion does not cover all current programs available for occupational therapy practitioners to contribute to the well-being of aging adults.

Independent Living

Most aging adults prefer to live independently in a familiar environment (Siebert, 2003). Independent living is defined as having and exercising control over choices of where and how to live, including choosing meaningful life roles and reaching independent decisions about managing activities of daily living, instrumental activities of daily living, and social interactions. These choices are made independently or with minimal dependence upon others (Freiden & Cole, 1985). The independent living model includes modifying inaccessible environments as well as removing barriers such as negative attitudes of others (Bowen, 2001). Independent living has been enhanced by universal design, which focuses on making home and public spaces usable for persons of all abilities and ages, and helps provide aging adults with attractive spaces and products, allowing them to continue to pursue valued activities.

Occupational therapy practitioners and other healthcare providers have collaborated in addressing desires of older adults to stay in their homes by evaluating home environments and making recommendations for cost-effective modifications (Cornerly, Elfenbein & Macias-Moriarty, 2001; Stark, 2004). The focus of most efforts to facilitate "aging in place" includes assessing the home for safety and identifying environmental and architectural barriers within it. Other collaborative efforts have included assessing and removing barriers in the community so that persons with disabilities and aging adults can participate in community life during routine activities such as banking, food shopping, and socializing (Reid, 2004; Oliver, Chiu, Marshall & Goldsilver, 2003; Petersson, Fisher & Hemingsson, 2007). The national aging network serves health and wellness needs of aging adults in communities throughout the United States. Offering many services including health promotion, congregate and home delivered meals, transportation, counseling, adult day care, and elder abuse prevention, these local networks are designed to keep aging adults in their homes and communities (Orr, Rogers & Scott, 2006).

Students engaged in community service have implemented many "aging in place" programs. Programs that make it easier for aging adults to stay in their own homes provide students with opportunities to apply concepts learned in the classroom to a community experience working with an older population. Private practices, however, also provide home evaluation and modifications as a professional service paid for by aging adults planning to stay in their homes. As the population ages, many people with the financial means to provide themselves with a preferred lifestyle will seek out those who can help them maintain their independence. Although it would seem that third-party payers would value the reduced cost of maintaining people in their own homes rather than in institutions, the U.S. healthcare system has not been aggressive in paying for these services. Fortunately, private payment is possible for a large segment of the aging population (Peters, 2005).

Kitchens can be modified or rearranged to be safe and functional so that as individuals experience disability or diminished capacity, they can still perform valued activities. Home exteriors can be evaluated for barriers such as steps and uneven ground. Once barriers have been identified, a therapist can collaborate with the older adult to determine what changes are to be made, where to locate products, and to arrange for installation. An occupational therapy practitioner working with a subcontractor to make a home more accessible may facilitate home modifications.

Evaluation of a home includes identifying safety hazards to prevent falls. Falls are a major concern of older people living in their own homes. L. Knecht-Sabres (personal communication November 29, 2005) states that approximately one-third of all persons over age 65 living in the community fall each year. By age 80, about half of elders living in the community fall. Falls are the leading cause of death and disability among those aged 65 or older, and most falls go undetected until they lead to serious injury. Many elders do not report falling in their home because they fear that a fall will mean they will be forced to leave their homes, and will lose control over their lives.

L. Knecht-Sabres (personal communication November 29, 2005), recognized that falls lead to significant healthcare costs and developed a fall prevention program. She proposes assessment of a person at risk for falls to include observation of the person engaged in occupational performance in his home environment. Close (2003) found that a single medical evaluation, followed by a referral to an occupational therapy practitioner for assessment of environmental factors that may contribute to falls, prevented first falls and produced a significant decrease in the number of further falls. People who have been assessed for risk of falling are likely to follow the suggestions made (Clemson et al., 2004). In addition to observing the environment to eliminate objects or conditions that may contribute to falls, evaluation of the person takes into consideration the following: vision and hearing, depression, dizziness, fear of falling, urinary incontinence, and cognition. These are all factors known to contribute to falls in the elderly. Intervention recommendations made to an aging adult are specific to a person's individual needs and preferences.

Berg, Hines & Allen (2002) found that only 10 percent of persons living at home and using a wheelchair for mobility had an environment suited to their functional limitations. As a result many wheelchair users experienced injurious falls. The most helpful modifications for preventing falls were in bathrooms and kitchens, and also included widening doors and hallways, adding railings, and making doors easier to open. Any one of these modifications to the home decreased the prevalence of injurious falls (Berg, Hines & Allen, 2002).

Caring for Caregivers

The majority of persons aging with dementia remain in their homes, cared for by family members. Often the family member providing care is himself aging and receives little assistance from others. Persons with dementia experience a continuum of diminished capacity in performing activities of daily living, instrumental activities of daily living, socialization, and control of body functions. They may engage in challenging behaviors such as emotional outbursts and wandering, and often resist care. Gitlin, Corcoran, Winter, Boyce & Marcus (1999) studied caregivers' abilities to sustain care during the course of the dementia of a loved one. They focused on occupational therapy interventions including home modification and use of strategies to manage the person with dementia. They found that caregivers who were depressed were unlikely to follow through with either type of intervention. They also found that women caregivers were more likely to focus on the emotional aspects of care, while men caregivers tended to approach care more as an extension of their worker role. Although care burden is known to contribute to stress, depression, and physical illness, few health providers address the caregiver's needs (Greven, 2007). Occupational therapy practitioners working with older adults in community practice can remain observant for caregiver stress. Using a client centered model to address a caregiver's needs, and providing stress reduction and referral to support groups and community activities, may enable the caregiver to remain healthy and allow the client to remain at home.

Providing continuity of care from hospital to home, or among different service providers, may assist caregivers as well as those who are receiving care. An example from England describes maintaining aging adults in their homes after discharge from hospital by using a multidisciplinary home care team that reduces need for residential care. Sending a client home from hospital with this care was less costly than sending an aging person home without home care, and provided a cost benefit to a national health insurance program that needed to constrain overall healthcare cost (Healy, Victor, Thomas & Seargeant, 2002). Collaboration among disciplines to provide continuity of care between hospital and home led to decreased institutional care for those who received the service, further supporting the value of community care.

A Story from Practice

While I worked in London, one of my clients who had for years received community care for mental illness reached her 65th birthday, the point at which her care was to be transferred to an elder care team. The elder care team used a holistic approach to treatment, comprehensively evaluating physical, cognitive, and emotional well-being and planning intervention to address special needs of aging adults. Together with the leader of the community elder care team to whom I would transfer my client, I planned a joint visit to facilitate my client's transition of care. During the visit I had an opportunity to see how elder care in the community effectively managed the special needs of an aging adult. Physical and mental health were coordinated by a single team specialized in geriatric care including a physician, a nurse, a social worker, and an occupational therapist. If the client needed hospitalization, both physical and mental health care was provided at a single location staffed by health professionals who specialized in geriatric medicine. The continuity of care between hospital and community was reassuring to the client and her family. They knew that when she required care, those who provided it would be familiar with her physical and psychological health needs.

Although this example comes from a single-payer universal healthcare system outside the United States, cost saving resulting from integration of services across institutions and different service providers has relevance for persons receiving health care paid for by Medicare, a national health organization. Providing a community service that links clients and their families with multiple service providers and agencies may be an opportunity for occupational therapy practitioners working with aging adults in the community to enhance service outcomes and quality of life for both clients and family members.

Maintaining Physical Abilities

Physical activities to maintain flexibility and strength become even more important as people age. Exercise is recommended to prevent falls, and aging adults may be directed to a variety of exercise programs in the community. Tai Chi has been found to be very helpful for preventing falls in the elderly, who experience a 48 percent reduction in falls after practicing this form of exercise (Carter, Kannus & Khan, 2001; Painter & Elliot, 2004).

Aquatics therapy is another example of a program that helps aging adults effectively maintain physical activity despite aging and painful joints. Most physical and occupational therapists who have developed these and similar programs collaborated with local recreation or community service facilities that already included a swimming pool. Some therapists have specifically designed water therapy programs that include pool and changing facilities to accommodate persons with disabilities. Water therapy is used for rehabilitation, general conditioning, and weight reduction because swimming or walking in the water has been shown to reduce the stress on joints that would otherwise occur during walking or exercise activities on land (Gappmaier, Lake, Nelson & Fisher, 2006). Swimming and water gymnastics have proven to be well tolerated by persons with cardiovascular disease, which may be found among aging adults (Schmid et al., 2007). One of the most common problems of aging is the pain of arthritis, which reduces activity level in older adults. Activities in water reduce pain while providing the benefits of an improved overall physical condition (Vaht, Birkenfeldt & Ubner, 2008; Kuphal, Fibuch & Taylor, 2007). While swimming and water based rehabilitation programs are available for persons of all ages and abilities, occupational therapy practitioners can collaborate with existing community programs to develop and provide water conditioning and therapy specifically for aging adults, allowing them an important opportunity to maintain physical ability and wellness.

Occupational therapy practitioners also are engaged in collaboration with community organizations to develop and implement a variety of other exercise and relaxation programs to accommodate the changing physical abilities of aging adults. Yoga, tai chi, Pilates, and dance activities may be offered to all residents of a community through a recreation center, but many of these activities are directed toward a young and generally well-conditioned population. Aging adults, although interested in these activities, may not participate due to inability to keep up with younger participants. Occupational therapy practitioners can adapt these activities for persons of differing abilities and incorporate other valued occupations, such as socialization, to keep aging adults engaged in physical activity. The recent emphasis placed on containing the cost of aging though engagement in a healthier lifestyle has increased the importance of developing exercise programs specifically designed for an older population (Timmons, 2008).

Assisted Living in the Community

Assisted living provides an aging adult privacy and an autonomous lifestyle while at the same time making assistance available as needed for certain activities. Assisted living is an option usually chosen for a person aging with a disability or one who can no longer care for herself independently. Assisted living arrangements are often chosen and made by family members. An aging adult in an assisted living facility has her own apartment or small home adjacent to others also occupied by persons needing some assistance with daily living. People living in these arrangements do not require nursing care but some may need help with meals, transportation, or recreational activities. They may also choose to pay for additional services such as occupational, physical, or speech therapy; personal care assistance; or housekeeping services. The advantage of assisted living versus a long-term care or nursing facility for aging adults is the independence allowed in choice of activities and the timing of those activities. By living in their own apartments, residents can choose when to have a meal or what they will eat. They can sleep and engage in other activities according to their own schedule, as opposed to the schedule of an institution. They can enter their own homes at will, close the door, and be alone when they choose, which is often impossible in an institution. For family members, assisted living offers peace of mind that their elder is not alone, is being monitored by staff of the living community, and can get help immediately if needed.

Occupational therapy practitioners may provide more traditional rehabilitation services to persons in assisted living accommodations through a home health care agency (Fisher, Atler & Potts, 2007). Some occupational therapy practitioners, however, are consulting with assisted living communities to provide activities that promote healthy aging or to provide home modifications that increase resident safety. Activities to promote wellness and health include fall prevention, exercise, stress reduction, and other programs that meet the interests and needs of clients. Such programs contribute greatly to maintenance of the more independent lifestyle desired by aging adults (McPhee & Johnson, 2000; Scott et al., 2001). Assisted living centers are being developed to accommodate baby boomers' consumer preferences along with their desires for independence and comfort. The residents of these facilities can and will pay privately for services that they believe will enhance their lifestyles.

Adult Day Care

Adult day care programs are community based and offer a variety of services to aging adults and their families. These programs are especially helpful to the children or spouse of a person with dementia or other condition who cannot safely be left alone during the day. Fuhr, Martinez, and Williams (2008) estimate that by 2020 there will be 157 million persons living with chronic health conditions who will be receiving informal care from family members. Day care programs offer either daily or occasional respite care to this large and unpaid workforce. Participants in adult day care continue to live at home, usually with family members, but are safely supervised during the day. The support day care offers for family members allows them to engage in leisure and social activities during the day or just to have some time to care for their own needs while being assured that their elder is safe and cared for. This support helps reduce the feelings of depression that some family members develop while they care for elders at home, isolated from activities and friends they once enjoyed. For many caregivers still working, adult day care allows them to continue to engage in full-time employment outside the home. Some employers sponsor or help pay for adult day care as a benefit of employment, recognizing that when their employees are not worrying about the safety of their aging family member they are free to be more productive workers.

Day care programs offer activities to engage participants in socialization and mental or physical stimulation. Some programs assist clients with self-care, such as bathing or other hygiene activities, so that families do not have to provide this assistance at home. Meals are usually provided during the day. Medical or rehabilitation services may also be provided to participants. Adult day care is intended to provide services that maximize the aging adult's independence; provide support, respite, and education to family members; and encourage socialization with staff members and other persons attending the program. Adult day care uses an interdisciplinary approach to accomplish its purpose, and often includes nursing, social work, activities therapy, and occupational therapy. Many adult day care programs are operated by non-healthcare providers in consultation with health professionals as needed.

Occupational therapy practitioners who participate in adult day care programs offer a unique perspective because of their knowledge regarding human development throughout the life span and the changing roles and interests of aging adults. They are skilled in the assessment of a person's physical, emotional, and cognitive abilities and can identify activities that are meaningful for each person. As a consultant, an occupational therapy practitioner can design activities for groups of participants in the program or modify activities for persons with special needs. Some occupational therapy practitioners direct adult day care programs, others serve as consultants, and some provide traditional rehabilitation services at adult day care centers within the community.

While many day care programs are designed for aging adults with a disability or dementia, other adult day programs are designed for well elders who want to maintain their health and well-being. These programs may offer a variety of activities such as exercise, yoga or tai chi, games, arts and crafts, meals, and group outings to films, plays, museums, or other cultural events. Participants choose which activities to attend, and transportation may be provided by the community. There may be a cost to participate in the activities or they may be free, depending on the agency offering the program. These programs strive to keep aging adults engaged in the community, keep them physically and mentally active, and allow them to remain socially engaged with others to enhance overall health and well-being. Engagement in this type of program is especially beneficial for aging adults who need to identify new interests to occupy time previously spent in paid employment, or who want to establish new relationships as old friends relocate or die.

Driving Assessment of Aging Adults

One area of practice certain to expand in the United States is driving assessment of aging adults. The number of older drivers is expected to double between 1990 and 2030 (Unsworth, 2007). Occupational therapy has responded to this opportunity by developing specialty certification in driving and community mobility (Stav & Lieberman, 2008). Practice guidelines for driving and community mobility for older adults are available through the American Occupational Therapy Association (AOTA, 2007). AOTA has collaborated with the American Society on Aging, American Association of

Retired Persons (AARP), and the Automobile Association of America (AAA) in a "car fit" program that suggests car modification or driving services (Strzlecki, 2008). Training courses are available for therapists who wish to apply their professional skills and knowledge to developing driving assessment programs and obtaining certification to offer these services to their communities.

As aging occurs, some physical and cognitive abilities naturally decline, yet aging adults are reluctant to give up driving because to them this means giving up their independence. In isolated or rural areas with large open spaces and poor public transportation, the car is a means of survival and is associated with freedom to choose and be independent. Getting a driver's license is a rite of passage for teenagers, and being able to move about on one's own becomes a way of life. Asking an aging adult to stop driving is an emotional and disruptive event. Family members may have difficulty making a decision about how safe their elder is behind the wheel. This can lead to conflict and counterproductive behaviors within the family.

A Story from Practice

A parent of a friend has had several minor car accidents in the past year. She often forgets where she has parked her car when she drives to the supermarket, and gets very anxious about not being able to find her way home. Her family has asked her to stop driving her car but she has refused. She explains that she will lose her independence if she cannot drive. She says she doesn't know how she will get food or go to the doctor if she can't drive herself to these locations. She says she will be unable to have lunch with her friends if she cannot drive to the restaurant. She says that if her family takes her car keys away, she will not speak to them again. This puts the family in a difficult position. They feel that their mother cannot safely drive her car, that she could have an accident and hurt herself or someone else, but they don't want their mother to be angry with them if they take her car from her.

This is a common situation for many families. In many cities public transportation is either nonexistent or inadequate; residents drive their own cars to wherever they need or want to go. Where public transportation is available, it may be inconvenient or not easily accessible to aging adults. Buses may run according to a schedule better suited to workers traveling to and from a job and less well-suited to elders needing to get to and from social events or doctor's appointments. Some agencies provide transportation for a fee, but many elders feel this is inconvenient and limits their ability to go where they want when they want.

While performing a driving assessment, an occupational therapy practitioner will look at the person's total functional ability (Hunt & Arbesman, 2008). She can evaluate an older adult's physical ability to sense stimuli in the environment, such as sound or sight, and determine if this ability is impaired. In many cases sensory impairments such as sight and hearing can be corrected with glasses or a hearing aid. An occupational therapy practitioner can evaluate an individual's physical strength and response times for safety in driving. She can perform a cognitive assessment to determine if the person can identify hazards and respond safely. She also will evaluate whether the client's functional abilities are compatible with driving safely in the community. Hunt and Arbesman (2008) point out that classroom performance, while promoting a sense of competence, does not necessarily transfer to driving safely in the community. Modifications may be made to a car and compensatory techniques taught to the aging adult that will allow her to continue driving safely (Arbesman & Pellerito, 2008).

If a person cannot continue driving safely however, or is safe only under specific conditions, the specially trained and certified occupational therapy practitioner will state this recommendation to the aging adult (Unsworth, 2007). By working collaboratively with a client to help him accept his limitations regarding safe driving, the therapist empowers him to make additional decisions by identifying ways to maintain independence without driving. In some cases, driving may still be possible but with restrictions to daylight hours or use of adaptive devices. In addition, participation in therapy may be required to improve skills needed for safe driving (Poole, Chaudry & Jay, 2008).

Assessment by an occupational therapy practitioner allows the aging adult's family members to support their loved one rather than anger him by saying he cannot drive based solely on their beliefs that his driving is dangerous. When family relationships become strained in a power struggle over who can drive, it is advantageous to seek out an evaluation by an impartial person who will be able to make recommendations for safe driving.

Although assessing safe driving ability is a fairly new community practice for occupational therapy practitioners, it is a practice for which they are uniquely qualified because they can evaluate all dimensions of functional performance required for the task of driving. By offering to evaluate driving safety, occupational therapy practitioners contribute to the safety of the entire community by verifying that a driver can safely operate a car. As with other areas of occupational therapy practice, this will grow as the population ages. A time may come when aging adults will be required to undergo driving assessments to continue to hold a driver's license beyond a specific age, or when certain medical conditions apply to the driver.

CHAPTER SUMMARY

Opportunities to practice in the community with aging adults will increase over coming years. People are living longer and want to continue to engage in activities they find meaningful and pleasurable. Some will desire, or be required, to continue in the paid workforce; others will want to learn new skills or will increase their physical activity to maintain health. Aging adults may need assistance in adapting the environment to their changing physical needs. Families will seek assistance in caring for parents and partners who have dementia or other disabling conditions. A significant number of aging adults will be able to afford to pay for these services independent of health insurance.

While some areas of practice with aging adults have been identified in this section, the future of working with this population may contain hidden opportunities. Today, those entering their final third of a usual life span are deviating from previous generations in many ways. They are living to be older. They have experienced more transitions in work and social life than their predecessors. They are more assertive in stating what they want and expect from others in relationship to their own needs and desires. While many aging adults appear to be in exceptionally good physical condition, another group of adults is aging with poor health as a result of lifestyle choices. Obesity and smoking have led them to develop cardiovascular, respiratory, and joint diseases that are disabling and chronic.

In the future, occupational therapy practitioners will collaborate with aging adults to develop community programs yet to be defined. We can expect a continuing need for rehabilitation services for persons with chronic disability and disease, which will result in increased healthcare costs. Opportunities will also exist, however, to provide services directed toward wellness. These services can be expected to decrease overall healthcare costs, and will not be paid for through health insurance. While occupational therapy practitioners have traditionally been associated with health care as a medical profession, they have the knowledge and skills to provide non-healthcare related services. As the costs of health care become one of the greatest challenges of the future, occupational therapy may prove to be one of the most cost-effective services available to prevent or reduce medical expenses.

LEARNING ACTIVITIES

Most people define successful aging as the ability to continue the tasks of adulthood. Physical and economic challenges may alter plans made by aging adults at an earlier stage of life. Adapting to challenges provides community practice opportunities for occupational therapy practitioners who have the skills, knowledge, and preference for working with aging adults.

1. Retirement is most often associated with a particular age specified by government when one may receive Social Security benefits. Describe how economic factors are challenging this understanding.
2. Some aging adults never intend to retire from paid employment either because they enjoy their job or have no other means of support. What might a community practice designed to help aging workers remain effective in their jobs look like?
3. Consider the aging adult who has suddenly been assigned as the legal guardian of young children. What needs might this caregiver encounter while fulfilling this responsibility? What skills and knowledge might an occupational therapy practitioner bring to addressing these challenges?
4. What community organizations or services in your community might provide opportunity for collaboration with an occupational therapy practitioner in addressing needs of aging adults?
5. Visit a community center or agency serving aging adults and observe the physical, social, and psychological needs of clients. Relate interventions that could be provided by an occupational therapy practitioner to meet client needs within this center or agency.
6. Talk to one or two aging adults in your community about their performance patterns and concerns they may have about continuing valued occupations as they age. Collaborate in developing a list of interventions that could be provided by an occupational therapy practitioner to meet their needs and the needs of other aging adults in your community. Discuss which of these interventions they would pay for privately and how much they would pay if these services were offered.

REFERENCES

American Occupational Therapy Association (2007). Board and specialty certification. From www.aota.org/practitioners/profdev/certification.aspx.

Arbesman, M. & Pellerito, J.M. (2008). Evidence-based perspective on the effect of automobile-related modifications on the driving ability, performance and safety of older adults. *The American Journal of Occupational Therapy, 62* (2) 173–186.

Bass-Haugen, J., Henderson, M.L., Larson, B.A. & Matuska, K. (2005) Occupational issues of concern in populations. In C.C. Christiansen and C.M. Baum (Eds.) *Occupational therapy performance, participation and well-being.* (pp.166–187). Thorofare, NJ: Slack, Inc.

Berg, K., Hines, M. & Allen, S. (2002). Wheelchair users at home: Few modifications and many injurious falls. *Journal of Public Health, 92* (1) 48.

Bonder, B., Dal Bello-Haas, V. & Wagner, M.B. (2009). *Functional performance in older adults* (3rd ed.) Philadelphia, PA: F.A. Davis Co.

Bouck, C. (2008). Design for the ages. *Parks and Recreation, 43* (6) 62–66.

Bowen, R.E. (2001) Independent living programs. In M. Scaffa (Ed.) *Occupational therapy in community-based practice settings.* (pp. 173–187). Philadelphia, PA: F.A. Davis.

Bren, L. (2003). Alzheimer's: Searching for a cure. *FDA Consumer, 37* (4) 18.

Brown, C.A., McGuire, F.A. & Voelkl, J. (2008). The link between successful aging and serious leisure. *International Journal of Aging and Human Development, 66* (1) 73–95.

Bull, M.J. & McShane, R.E. (2008). Seeking what's best during transition to adult day health services. *Qualitative Health Research, 18* (5) 597–605.

Cajigal, S. (2008). One in eight baby boomers expected to develop AD. *Neurology Today, 8* (9) 20.

Carter, N., Kannus, P. & Khan, K. (2001). Exercise in the prevention of falls in older people: A systematic literature review examining the rationale and evidence. *Sports Medicine, 31,* 427–438.

Clemson, L., Cumming, R.G., Kendig, H., Swann, M., Heard, R. & Taylor, K. (2004). The effectiveness of a community-based program for reducing the incidence of falls in the elderly: A randomized trial. *Journal of the American Geriatrics Society, 52* (9) 1487–1494.

Close, J.C.T., Hooper, R., Glucksman, E., Jackson, S.H.D. & Swift, G.C. (2003). Predictors of falls in high risk populations: Results from the prevention of falls in elderly trial. *Emergency Medicine Journal, 20* (5) 421–425.

Cornerly, H., Elfenbein, P. & Macias-Moriarty, L. (2001). Interdisciplinary health promotion education for low income older adults. *Journal of Physical Therapy Education, 15* (2) 37–41.

Freedman, V.A., Martin, L.G., Schoeni, R.F. & Cornman, J.C. (2008). Declines in late life disability: The role of early and mid life factors. *Social Science and Medicine, 66* (7) 1588–1602.

Fisher, A.G., Atler, K. & Potts, A. (2007). Effectiveness of occupational therapy with frail community living older adults. *Scandinavian Journal of Occupational Therapy, 14* (4) 240–249.

Freiden, L. & Cole, J.A. (1985). Independence: The ultimate goal of rehabilitation with spinal cord injured persons. *American Journal of Occupational Therapy, 39* 734–739.

Fuhr, P., Martinez, B. & Williams, M. (2008). Research report. Caregivers with visual impairment: A preliminary study. *Journal of Visual Impairment & Blindness, 102* (2) 89–96.

Gappmaier, E., Lake, W., Nelson, A.G. & Fisher, A.G. (2006). Aerobic exercise in water versus walking on land: Effects on indices of fat reduction and weight loss in obese women. *Journal of Sports Medicine & Physical Fitness, 46* (4) 564–569.

Gitlin, L.N., Cocoran, M., Winter, L., Boyce, A. & Marcus, S. (1999). Predicting participation and adherence to home environmental intervention among family caregivers of persons with dementia. *Family Relations, 48,* 363–372.

Greven, C. (2007). Caring for the caregiver. *OT Practice, 12* (16) 25–26.

Haak, M., Fange, A., Horstmann, V. & Iwarsson, S. (2008). Two dimensions of participation in very old age and their relations for home and neighborhood environments. *The American Journal of Occupational Therapy, 62* (1) 77–86.

Healy, J., Victor, C.R., Thomas, A. & Seargeant, J. (2002). Professionals and post-hospital care for older people. *Journal of Interprofessional Care, 16* (1) 133–148.

Huguet, N., Kaplan, M.S. & Feeny, D. (2008). Socioeconomic status and health related quality of life among elderly people: Results from joint Canada/United States survey of health. *Social Science and Medicine, 66* (4) 803–810.

Hunt, L. & Arbesman, M. (2008). Evidence-based and occupational perspective of effective interventions for older clients that remediate or support improved driving performance. *The American Journal of Occupational Therapy, 62* (2) 136–148.

Koo, L.C. (1987). *Nourishment of life: Health in Chinese society*. Hong Kong: The Commercial Press, Ltd.

Kuphal, K.E., Fibuch, E.E. & Taylor, B.K. (2007). Extended swimming exercise reduces inflammatory and peripheral neuropathy pain in rodents. *Journal of Pain Management, 8* (12) 989–997.

Lau, A. & McKenna, K. (2001). Conceptualizing quality of life for elderly people with stroke. *Disability and Rehabilitation, 23* (6) 227–238.

McPhee, S.D. & Johnson, T. (2000). Program planning for an assisted living community. *Occupational Therapy in Health Care, 12* (2/3) 1–17.

Oliver, R., Chiu, T., Marshall, L. & Goldsilver, P. (2003). Home safety assessment and intervention practice. *International Journal of Therapy and Rehabilitation, 10* (4) 140–148.

Orr, A.L., Rogers, P. & Scott, J. (2006). Roundup: The complexities and connectedness of the public health and aging networks. *Journal of Visual Impairment & Blindness, 100*. Special supplement, pp. 874–877.

Painter, J. & Elliet, S. (2004). Developing and implementing a senior community based fall prevention and safety program. *Occupational Therapy in Health Care, 18* (3) 21–32.

Peters, T. (2005). *Re-imagine! Business excellence in a disruptive age*. London: Dorling Kindersley Ltd.

Peterson, I., Fisher, A.G., Hemmingsson, M.L. (2007). The client-clinician assessment protocol (C-CAP): Evaluation of its psychometric properties for use with people aging with disabilities in need of home modifications. *Occupational Therapy Journal of Research: Occupation, Participation & Health, 27* (4) 140–148.

Plassman, B.L., Langa, K.M., Fisher, G.G., Heeringa, S.G., Weir, D.R., Ofstedal, M.B., et al. (2008). Prevalence of cognitive impairment without dementia in the United States. *Annals of Internal Medicine, 148* (6) 427–434.

Poole, D., Chaudry, F. & Jay, W.M. (2008). Stroke and driving. *Topics in Stroke Rehabilitation, 15* (1) 37–41.

Reid, D. (2004). Accessibility and usability of the physical housing environment of seniors with stroke. *International Journal of Rehabilitation Research, 27* (3) 203–208.

Reyes-Ortiz, C.A., Pelaez, M., Koenig, H.G. & Mulligan, T. (2007). Religiosity and self-rated health among Latin American and Caribbean elders. *International Journal of Psychiatry in Medicine, 37* (4) 425–443.

Salloway, S., Feldman, H.H., Kandiah, N. & DeKosky, S.T. (2008). Expert review supplement. Next steps in Alzheimer's disease: Improvement in diagnosis and treatment. *CNS Spectrums: The International Journal of Neuropsychiatric Medicine 13* (3) 1–2.

Scott, A.H., Butin, D.N., Tewfik, D., Burkardt, A., Mandel, D. & Nelson, L. (2001). Occupational therapy as a means to wellness with the elderly. *Physical & Occupational Therapy in Geriatrics, 18* (4) 3–22.

Schmid, J.P., Noveanu, M., Morger, C., Gaillet, R., Capoferri, M., Anderegg, M. & Saner, H. (2007). Influence of water immersion, water gymnastics and swimming on cardiac output in patients with health failure. *Heart, 93* (6) 722–727.

Siebert, C. (2003). Aging I place: Implications for occupational therapy. *OT Practice, 8* (8) 16–20.

Stark, S. (2004). Removing environmental barriers in the homes of older adults with disabilities improves occupational performance. *Occupational Therapy Journal of Research, 24* (1) 32–39.

Stav, W.B., Arbesman, M. & Lieberman, D. (2008). Background and methodology of the older driver evidence-based systematic literature review. *The American Journal of Occupational Therapy, 62* (2) 130–135.

Stav, W.B. & Lieberman, D. (2008). From the desk of the editor. *The American Journal of Occupational Therapy, 62* (2) 127–129.

Strzelecki, M. (2008). Driving the profession. *OT Practice, 13* (5) 9,11.

Timmons, N. (2008, July 2). Bingo and patient back-up prove life-enhancing. *Financial Times*, p. 8.

Timmons, N. (2008, July 2). Growing ranks of the elderly add to age-old costs dilemma. *Financial Times*, p. 8.

Turner, J.A. (2008). Work options for older Americans. *Benefits Quarterly, 24* (3) 20–25.

Unsworth, C.A. (2007). Using social judgment theory to study occupational therapists' use of information when making driver licensing recommendations for older and functionally impaired adults. *The American Journal of Occupational Therapy, 61* (5) 493–502.

Vaht, M., Birkenfeldt, R. & Ubner, M. (2008). An evaluation of the effectiveness of the effect of differing length of spa therapy upon patients with osteoarthritis. *Complementary Therapies in Clinical Practice, 14* (1) 60–64.

Vallant, G. (2002). *Aging well.* Boston: Little Brown & Co.

Wang, C., Chan, C.L.W., Ng, S. & Ho, A.H.Y. (2008). The impact of spirituality on health related quality of life among Chinese older adults with vision impairments. *Aging and Mental Health, 12* (2) 267–275.

Chapter 6

Community Mental Health Practice

LEARNING OBJECTIVES

- Appreciate the historical context of community mental health practice.
- Explain cost efficacy of assertive outreach for persons with mental illness.
- Identify options for community mental health practice.

INTRODUCTION

Mental illness directly affects one in four Americans and indirectly affects many more family members, coworkers, and friends (NIMH, 2008). Mental illness may begin with a gradual decline in a person's abilities to perform routines of work, self-care, and leisure activities, or as a sudden crisis that is difficult to predict and manage (Roth & McCune, 2005). A crisis may be followed by medical evaluation and medication. A person who responds well to a prescribed medication may return home and resume his life roles, needing only periodic medical monitoring.

CHALLENGES OF MENTAL ILLNESS

Other persons diagnosed with mental illness have a more challenging future because they either do not respond well to medication or may choose not to take medication, allowing symptoms of their illness to continue. Not every person experiences relief of symptoms, even when alternative medicines are used. Many medications require a prolonged period of use before beneficial effects become apparent. This long waiting period causes many people to abandon medications before symptom relief can occur. Others find that side effects from medication are unpleasant and they are unwilling to continue taking the medicine even if it brings some relief of symptoms. When I worked in community mental health, many clients told me they discontinued their prescribed medicine because they did not like the way it made them feel. Some clients said they stopped taking medicine because they did not think they needed it anymore. Over time, people whose symptoms of mental illness continue may become socially isolated from family and friends, which can increase their stress levels and exacerbate symptoms of their illness, such as suicidal thoughts and tendencies (Russell & Lloyd, 2004).

People with persistent mental illness may be challenged to find and maintain paid employment. Many find their way into community mental health programs, become homeless, or enter the criminal justice system. Providing adequate services to enhance quality of life for persons with mental illness is challenging in the face of inadequate funding for services. Cottrell (2007) discusses federal initiatives designed to facilitate community integration of persons with mental illness, but these programs remain largely unfunded. Approximately half of all persons who are homeless are also mentally ill, and services directed toward homeless populations are not always equipped to handle persons with mental illness (Cottrell, 2007).

Services do exist to assist people with mental illness to function at their best possible levels in their communities, a goal of the New Freedom Initiative (2003). These services include community based day treatment and clubhouse and assertive outreach programs for people who either remain in their own homes or are homeless. These programs and others offer creative opportunities for occupational therapy practitioners interested in serving persons with mental illness in the community. Financing these programs, however, continues to be a challenge due to limited government resources and little incentive or ability to pay for these services privately.

HISTORICAL CONTEXT OF COMMUNITY MENTAL HEALTH

Mental health treatment began in the community, gradually became institution-based, and has now returned to the community. Before there were medical interventions, persons with mental illness lived at home with their families. If families were unable to provide care at home, they sent their ill family member to a community of persons with mental illness to be cared for by others (Paterson, 2002). Within these communities, members became self-sufficient by growing and preparing food, making their own clothing, and engaging in other activities needed to sustain themselves and others living there. Engaging in meaningful and purposeful activities allowed persons with mental illness, and those who cared for them, to become a mutually supportive community (Paterson, 2003; Schwartz, 2005).

As industrialization and urban living became economic realities, agrarian lifestyles that previously had accommodated persons with mental illness ceased to exist. Institutions were constructed to house people with symptoms of mental illness who were feared and misunderstood by others in the community. These institutions held few opportunities to engage in purposeful activities and few treatments to alleviate symptoms. Consequently, most people living in these institutions had bleak existences. Furthermore, most of these institutions were located away from major urban areas or isolated by high walls, keeping persons with mental illness largely out of sight and out of mind. People with mental illness were a unknown population and yet they were harshly judged because of their unusual behaviors, which were symptoms of their illness. In the middle of the twentieth century, psychotropic medicines began to be developed that could provide relief of some symptoms of mental illness (Schwartz, 2005). As more medications were developed, increasing numbers of people with mental illness were discharged from institutions. Deinstitutionalization was envisioned as a cost saving initiative, and occupancy rates fell as institutions discharged their patients into the community. Unfortunately, a lack of symptoms of mental illness did not mean that the illness was gone for good. In addition, not all persons discharged to their communities had sufficient skills to maintain themselves. Many former residents had never lived outside an institution. A great many of them had no home or family to whom they could return. In addition, funding for community based mental health programs was very limited.

Eventually the cost to operate aging psychiatric institutions for the few residents who remained exceeded the benefit the institution brought to a community. The institutions began closing many of their buildings, yet retained disproportionately large staffs to care for the remaining patients, many of whom were considered the most ill or dangerous to themselves or others. The buildings were old and needed repairs or costly renovations to remain safely in operation. These costs and poor environmental conditions led to closure of most of the remaining mental health institutions in the last half of the twentieth century (Stein & Cutler, 1998; Weissbrem-Padan et al., 2006). As a result, numerous programs were developed to transition the remaining residents of institutions into the community. Unfortunately, sufficient funding for programs that would have offered support and skills for community living was not forthcoming. Many discharged patients were unable to receive necessary services in their communities.

Institutional life can have a negative impact on successful transition to community living (Fisher & Hotchkiss, 2008). Surprisingly, it does not take very long for a person to become dependent on others to provide care. As this occurs, the skills a person may have once relied upon for community living begin to deteriorate.

A Story from Practice

A community mental health client was hospitalized suffering from depression. She had lived her entire life at home, successfully raising two children who were now adults and had left home to work and begin their own families. Her sister, who had been supportive of her living at home, had recently died. Over the next few months a pattern was established in which this client would rapidly improve and be sent home, only to return to the hospital within a day or two. Her family was concerned that each time she came home, she was able to do less for herself. When she returned to the hospital she participated in activities, took walks in the community, and was generally cheerful. I continually worked with this client and her daughter, planning for a successful homecoming. With repeated failures to stay at home, we began discussing supported housing so that she would not be alone in her large house and could have help when necessary. My client refused this suggestion, however, stating that she was capable of going home and staying there. During her periods of hospitalization she did not need to shop, cook, clean her home, attend to a schedule, or do anything she did not want to do. The staff who cared for her in the hospital enjoyed having her. Her skill at maintaining herself and her home deteriorated. During a hospital renovation project, she was moved to a different treatment unit and her new medical staff explained to her that she had become "institutionalized," relying on others for her care. She was discharged to supported housing where she would be taught once more to care for herself.

Occupational therapy practitioners possess skills and knowledge valuable to persons who need to learn how to live in the community. Assessment includes understanding a person's cognitive and physical abilities, how affect or mood influences performance, and environmental factors that support or challenge community living. Occupational therapy practitioners who work with hospitalized mental health clients usually focus on developing task and social skills, and increasing awareness of non-productive behaviors. Short-duration hospitalizations provide little time for addressing many aspects of community living. When mental health care is provided in the community, however, occupational therapy practitioners have more opportunity to teach or facilitate skills needed for clients to care for themselves outside of institutions. Community based treatment is the preferred approach to caring for persons with severe and chronic mental illness because it minimizes social isolation (Russell & Lloyd, 2004). Despite a call to transform the mental health delivery system to enable persons with mental illness to fully participate in community life, a lack of financial support to implement necessary services in the United States continues (Cottrell, 2007; Hogan, 2003).

ASSERTIVE OUTREACH IN MENTAL HEALTH

Assertive outreach is a service model designed to improve community living for persons with severe mental illnesses who are high service users. This model delivers services in homes or other living environments of clients with chronic and severe mental illness. It provides clients opportunities to develop self-worth, a meaningful social identity, and a social network within their natural environments rather than through a hospital or clinic (Gewurtz, Krupa, Eastabrook & Horgan, 2004). Community care provided by assertive outreach programs reduces costs of hospitalization and increases client satisfaction (Killaspy, Johnson, King & Bebbington, 2008; Peterson, Michael & Armstrong, 2006).

Assertive outreach has a rather long history beginning in Amsterdam in the 1930s. It was later implemented in France and the United States in the 1960s, where services were usually provided by outreach workers trained on the job to locate persons with mental illness and offer them support. These outreach workers generally lacked knowledge and skills to assess environmental stressors, or to help a client adapt to community living without avoiding more costly hospital care. As persons with mental illness in the United States and the United Kingdom were deinstitutionalized, assertive outreach became increasingly important. In the United States, the emphasis remained on locating persons with mental illness who were living on the streets and attempting to convince them to take medication. In the United Kingdom, assertive outreach emphasized maintaining people with chronic and severe mental illness in their homes, thus decreasing costs of hospital care. Assertive outreach services in the United Kingdom continue to be provided by skilled professionals including occupational therapists, social workers, nurses, and psychologists.

The purpose of assertive outreach is to maintain regular and frequent contact with a person with mental illness in order to monitor his clinical condition, provide effective intervention and rehabilitation, decrease any need for emergency hospitalization, and increase safety for the client and the community (Tyrer et al., 2007). Assertive outreach goes beyond case management because it allows a service provider to not only establish a therapeutic relationship with a client in the community, but also to provide intervention in times of need. The relationship between client and service provider appears to be the key to successful assertive outreach. Without assertive outreach, a person living with mental illness goes between clinic, hospital, and community, being seen by many different service providers, often trusting no one. With assertive outreach, one professional team member maintains regular contact with a client. The client can rely on this professional for help when needed. Since assertive outreach is provided within the community where the client lives, the service provider is not limited to traditional institutional boundaries but instead has flexibility in meeting client needs whenever they arise.

A Story from Practice

While working as an occupational therapist in the community, I discovered that a principal goal of most of my clients was maintaining their homes. Money management was a problem for clients and although we worked on this problem, utility bills often went unpaid. When a cutoff notice was received, or in some cases the electric service was stopped, there was immediate need to have heat and light in their homes restored. In order to be effective in keeping clients at home, I would need to respond promptly when they phoned in a state of crisis without heat, light, or use of electric appliances. Some clients needed me to arrange to have their utilities restored, but I was able to coach and support most clients as they negotiated with a utility company to make a payment and have services restored. Another occupational therapist working in the same environment told me that she believed working with utility companies was a social worker's job. She had decided to leave community practice because she said she was not doing what she considered to be occupational therapy. I saw things differently; for me, occupational therapy includes teaching clients whatever skills are necessary to keep them living in their own homes and helping them to avoid future crises.

Assertive outreach occurs at the client's preferred location. Most clients want the therapist to visit their home, a preference which has benefits for both the client and the therapist. The therapist gains a better understanding of problems and environmental barriers, and can be more responsive to demands of the client's home life. Living skills can be taught in the client's natural environment, empowering her to share control of intervention.

Persons who experience the best results from assertive outreach are those with unstable mental illness, who have poor relationships or minimal social engagement with others, or who face severe consequences, such as reinstitutionalization or potential to harm themselves or others, if they relapse. Assertive outreach also benefits people with severe and persistent mental illness who are caring for their children at home. Parenting is a role that remains important to a person with mental illness. Although some people with mental illness have their children removed from their care, with the support of assertive outreach services, a parent may continue to be effective in her role. Children prefer to stay with their parents and not be removed from home to be cared for by an agency or another person. When a child of a parent with mental illness develops behavior problems or begins to show symptoms of mental illness, treating the entire family group in community addresses concerns that affect the entire family (Darwish, Salmon, Ahuja & Steed, 2006).

A Story from Practice

The majority of my community mental health clients were parents. Their children ranged in age from a few months old through young adulthood. Most clients had two or more children they cared for while managing a severe and persistent mental illness.

Helping them cope on a daily basis included educating them about discipline and setting limits on a child's behavior, demonstrating and coaching effective communication with teachers and school personnel, facilitating understanding of developmental stages and age-related changes in their children, and reassuring them when they did a good job of parenting.

One challenging client lived with her two teenagers who had serious school truancy problems. These teenagers were frequently not attending school, claiming they were physically ill or having difficulty with teachers or peers. Often they left home in the morning but failed to attend school. This upset their mother because she feared the consequences of her children's truancy. Parents who allowed their children to engage in excessive absence from school were held responsible for their children's behavior and could be fined. More serious actions were implied if the truancy did not cease. My client was terribly afraid that this meant her children would be taken from her. She knew a mother whose babies had been placed in care because she was mentally ill and unable to care for her children safely. After reminding my client that she had been successfully parenting her children through to adolescence, and reassuring her that her children would not be taken from her, we were able to begin discussions with school personnel to find solutions to her children's chronic truancy.

Assertive outreach is ideal for persons not engaged with other services or for people with a history of poor compliance with treatment. This includes persons with a variety of mental illnesses such as bipolar affective disorder, schizophrenia, and borderline personality disorders. People with these illnesses have difficulty establishing and maintaining relationships, they have poor insight and judgment, and they may be at risk of harming themselves or others. Many of these people also may have a history of poor compliance with medication (Tam & Law, 2007).

Assertive outreach includes medical management as one component of treatment. Although taking prescribed medications is desirable, it is not required of a client unless neglecting to do so results in danger of harm to self or others (Tan & Law, 2007). The side effects of medication can be regularly monitored while the person remains at home. Community intervention focuses on all aspects of occupational performance with the client determining what she needs. Clients are seen frequently, usually once a week or more, so that their needs can be addressed as they change. Home visits sometimes require persistence on the part of the service provider. There is no guarantee the client will be home or will answer the door at the appointed time.

An occupational therapy practitioner providing assertive outreach must address all areas of living. Housing may be stable for most clients, but some will require assistance in finding a home or moving. Homeless people receiving assertive outreach usually identify housing, either temporary or permanent, as their primary concern. Some homeless people, however, prefer not to use temporary housing or shelters, as they mistrust others living there. Providing food, clothing, hygiene supplies, and blankets while working on an alternative housing arrangement is the responsibility of an outreach therapist. Management of financial benefits provided by the government or social service agencies is a challenge. Most clients live at or below the poverty level and have great difficulty meeting their basic needs on their income. Productivity is important to clients; even if they are unable to maintain a paying job, they want to engage in volunteer work or meaningful leisure activities. Some clients need help with personal hygiene; other clients may have difficulty interacting with others. Finding opportunities for socialization is important because social activities enhance the quality of life for a person with mental illness (Eklund, 2006).

A Story from Practice

A client stayed in her apartment most of the time, and told me she was bored. I asked her what she would like to do and she said "cook." This client was a woman of few words and poor social skills. I began to describe a variety of options for participating in cooking activities in the community. She decided to try a cooking group at a center serving persons with mental illness, and we arranged to visit the center together. Before she attended the cooking activity, I wanted to verify that she could locate the center, reach it on her own, and be familiar with the building and at least one of the staff members working there. We visited the center together and my client said she was comfortable with the place and could get there by herself for the next scheduled cooking activity.

On my next home visit to this client, I asked if she had enjoyed the cooking group and she told me she did not cook. She said she had gone to the center an hour before the cooking group was scheduled to begin and finding no one in the kitchen, had gone home. I asked her if she wanted me to go with her to the next cooking group at the center and she said no. I mentioned another cooking group that met in the evenings to prepare dinner. The client and I visited the place where dinner was to be held, talked to one of the sponsors of the event, and planned to attend the event together. The evening of the dinner, I met my client at her home and we took the bus to the location where dinner was to occur. I stayed for the entire evening, cooked, ate, and cleaned up alongside my client, facilitating her socialization with staff and other participants. After dinner, as we waited at the bus stop to return to our own homes, my client said she liked the dinner and was going to attend the next time it was held and that I did not need to go with her.

My client continued to attend the dinner activity—not every time it was held, but occasionally. Her choice to attend or not was based on the dinner menu and what she liked to eat. As a result of her success with the dinner activity, she identified other interests and gradually began to spend more time engaged in community activities with others.

This story illustrates that empowering a client to choose an activity and then become independent while engaged in it is linked to mastery of social integration (Eklund, 2007).

At every assertive outreach visit a service provider assesses, through observation and interview, the client's personal appearance, reported sleep patterns, changes in mood, irritability or hostility, compliance with medication, financial concerns, the condition of the home, and evidence of drug or alcohol use. When a problem in any of these areas is identified, the service provider can immediately begin work with the client to solve the problem. If the client is hostile or obviously using alcohol or drugs, the service provider must assess her own safety and either end the visit or request help if needed. If the client is not taking prescribed medication, the service provider will explain the purpose of medication and ask why it has not been taken. Side effects are the most common reason for noncompliance with medication. The service provider may facilitate the client's discussion of medication concerns with his psychiatrist. If a client has run out of medication, the service provider can assist the client to obtain more. Often while helping a client solve one problem, an occupational therapist will discover other problems that can also be addressed.

A Story from Practice

A client who had consistently complied with medication told me he was feeling badly because he had not had his medicine for two days. When I asked why, he said he had stopped going out and could not get to the pharmacy to pick up the medicine. I phoned his physician who arranged for me to pick up the prescribed medications and deliver them to the client. The next month, this client had once more run out of medication. Again I phoned his physician and discussed the situation. The physician told me there was a pharmacy that would deliver the medications if the client would phone them and request delivery. My client had no phone so I had him use my cell phone to call the pharmacy and arrange delivery of his medicine. During the same visit, we began the process of having a phone installed in my client's home so that he could once again independently manage his medication.

When working with clients in the areas of personal hygiene and instrumental activities of daily living, a service provider must be careful not to impose her standards on a client. On the other hand, some clients do not exhibit skills for safe independent living because they have never acquired skills for instrumental activities of daily living. Sorting out whether a skill has been learned and discarded, or has never been learned and should become a focus of intervention, influences a therapeutic relationship between client and occupational therapy practitioner.

A Story from Practice

A student was engaged in teaching simple cooking skills to a formerly homeless man in his new apartment. This was his first experience of independent living and he had not previously learned meal preparation, a skill that was required for him to remain in his apartment. When it was time to clean up after cooking, the client ran the dirty dishes and utensils under water and left them to dry. The student asked the client if he had used detergent to wash his dishes in the past, and he told her he had never washed dishes before, his mother had done this. For the next visit with this client, the student brought dishwashing detergent and taught him how to wash his dishes and safely clean up after preparing food.

COMMUNITY MENTAL HEALTH CENTERS

Partial hospitalization programs include day treatment in which a client attends a community center during the day and returns to his own home at night. These services may be offered in a hospital or a community center; location is less important than program format. Most of these programs offer therapy groups similar to those provided to hospitalized persons, in which participants can address specific problems they are having with community living. Day treatment programs for adolescents include school sessions, while day treatment for adults includes other types of productive and leisure activities. Advantages of day treatment programs include the cost savings that result from not having to provide overnight hospitalization and being able to integrate the client with his family and community during treatment. Although partial hospitalization programs are managed by hospitals, day treatment programs may also be sponsored by other community organizations. Day treatment programs are equally useful for persons with mental illness living in rural communities, where a low density of clients makes assertive outreach programs less cost-effective (Meyer & Morrissey, 2007).

One therapist described her work in a partial hospitalization program in an urban community mental health center. The clients she worked with had severe and chronic mental illness and most lived at or below the poverty level. She provided occupational therapy services that engaged clients in producing, marketing, and selling greeting cards. While working, her clients also learned social, cognitive, and prevocational skills. She said she was rewarded for her work by expressions of appreciation from her clients for the services they received. She said that without her program many clients would otherwise not have the means to participate in meaningful activities because they could not afford the cost of community activities. Although some of the clients came to the day program with some hesitancy due to their past experiences or symptoms of mental illness, they were able to build a sense of rapport with each other and relationships of trust with staff members.

The clubhouse model of care is an opportunity for occupational therapy practitioners to work collaboratively with clients to build skills for community living. This model of treatment is reminiscent of very early mental health communities in which clients and their caregivers lived together and were self-supporting. Although current clubhouse programs are not required to be self-supporting, everyone who is part of the program collaborates in the work of the club. Club membership is designed to connect persons with mental illness to their community (Scheinholz, 2001).

Responsibilities of membership include regular attendance and participation in activities that sustain the club. Many clubhouse programs offer some type of paid employment for their members, such as assembly of materials needed by local businesses or preparation of mailings for organizations. This work is arranged through a contract between the business or agency involved and the clubhouse. Some of the money made goes to clubhouse operations and some goes to the clubhouse members who do the work. In addition to contract work, clubhouses generally prepare and serve meals to members or to others in the community. Clubhouse members shop for food, prepare and serve the meal, and clean up afterwards. The activities provided by the clubhouse give members an opportunity to socialize and increase their competence to manage their community living.

An occupational therapy practitioner who works in a clubhouse is considered a member with the same responsibilities and privileges as all of the other members. The philosophy behind clubhouse programs is that each member contributes to the best of his or her ability; there is no hierarchy of roles because all roles are considered essential to making the clubhouse work. An occupational therapy practitioner may utilize professional skills and knowledge to facilitate planning, shopping, and meal preparation, or to teach prevocational and vocational skills to those working in paid employment. Task modification or teaching compensatory techniques helps clients succeed in their work.

WORKING WITH PEOPLE WHO ARE HOMELESS

Some people with mental illness find themselves without a place to live. Their illness may make it difficult for them to find and keep jobs to support themselves, and they may lack family support to provide them with a home. Government restrictions on welfare and disability benefits often contribute to homelessness; not all people who are homeless are diagnosed with mental illness (Herzburg & Finlayson, 2001). It is best not to categorize people who are homeless, because an unexpected job loss and difficult economic pressures can render anyone homeless in a relatively short period of time. Searching for another job may be a long and difficult process, especially if there are few jobs and many potential workers available in the community. Over time, an unemployed person may become discouraged and depressed and may begin using alcohol or drugs to numb his feelings of despair. Eventually, he will have used all of his savings and be unable to provide for basic needs such as food and housing. So although mental illness may precipitate homelessness, homelessness may also precipitate mental illness.

Most communities have programs for persons who are homeless. Some of these programs specifically serve people with a diagnosis of mental illness; other programs serve anyone who finds himself homeless. Some programs are gender specific and some care for entire families. Programs may provide temporary housing or send staff out into the community to provide services to clients who choose to continue living on the streets. The goal of most of these programs is to help homeless persons meet their basic needs for shelter or food.

Other programs offer assistance to clients searching for employment by teaching skills for community re-entry or improving self-care. Often these programs are sponsored by state or federal governments, or by local non-profit organizations. The services provided by programs for homeless people frequently reflect the sponsorship of the program. Most programs for homeless people cannot afford to hire an occupational therapy practitioner because they operate on very lean budgets, but they may hire an occupational therapy practitioner as a consultant or offer clinical education opportunities to students. Occupational therapy interventions may include support and skills for finding a place to live, finding and keeping a job, and providing opportunities to engage in activities that contribute to improved self-esteem. Consultative services may include program development and skills training for others who will provide direct service to clients.

As a direct service provider, occupational therapy practitioners have skills and knowledge to empower people to overcome negative effects of mental illness while living in the community (Mitchell & Jones, 2004). Youngstrom (2000) describes an occupational therapist utilizing the Canadian Occupational Performance Model to identify client strengths and meaningful occupations, establishing client centered goals and developing intervention plans to achieve the goals. Working with homeless people provides direct service opportunities, including group activities in which clients practice interpersonal skills while learning time and money management. Occupational therapy practitioners may also serve as case managers in programs for homeless people (Hafez, 2000).

As a consultant, an occupational therapy practitioner may collaborate with other service providers by suggesting interventions, such as skills training, to help clients maintain themselves or their homes. For example, an occupational therapist worked with a case manager to assess a client's living environment and made suggestions for helping him organize and clean his living space, reducing his risk of losing his home.

> ## A Story from Practice
>
> *An occupational therapist began working as a consultant in a homeless shelter and then assumed the role of case manager. As a case manager, she was assigned clients with whom she was to help establish and achieve specific goals. She met with clients individually and frequently to assist them with problem solving and accessing needed services. She helped her clients with finances, housing, work, leisure, medication management, and any other skills required for them to remain in the community. As a case manager, this occupational therapist had ongoing therapeutic relationships with her clients and assisted them as they encountered difficulties maintaining their community living environments. She also coached them to engage in community activities, such as leisure and paid or volunteer work.*

Many opportunities exist for occupational therapy practitioners to work with persons with mental illness in their communities. Providing direct or consultative services to supported housing programs, vocational rehabilitation programs, foster parent or parent support programs, and home care programs are all possibilities for therapists wanting to work in the community. While some programs have resources to employ an occupational therapy practitioner, many mental health programs have difficulty managing their lean budgets as non-profit organizations. There are, however, many organizations serving persons with mental illness that would welcome the voluntary efforts of occupational therapy practitioners to organize and provide programs that engage people in purposeful and meaningful activities to benefit the community.

CHAPTER SUMMARY

Community treatment of persons with severe and chronic mental illness allows them to remain part of their communities. Occupational therapy practitioners can provide skills for living by creating an accepting and supportive environment. Working in the community with persons with mental illness provides challenge and satisfaction to a practitioner who enjoys working with a variety of people in unique environments. While working in this area of practice, an occupational therapy practitioner will appreciate that client needs drive services provided and not use "role blurring" as an excuse to avoid some aspects of service. The ability to remain safe, confident, and flexible in meeting with clients in their homes is important to successful practice. Working collaboratively with clients and other service providers through periods of stress is essential. Most occupational therapy practitioners working in community mental health find themselves the only occupational therapy practitioner on their teams or in their programs. Finding colleagues with whom to consult and share ideas is important to maintaining professional identity in this practice. Although occupational therapy practitioners have been working in community mental health for many years, there continue to be many opportunities to expand our services and contribute positively to the lives of persons living with severe and chronic mental illness.

LEARNING ACTIVITIES

1. The Community Mental Health Act, a government program to discharge many people with chronic mental illness from institutions, was not accompanied by federal funding to provide alternative programs for these people to become integrated into community life. Identify occupational therapy interventions that may assist persons who have little experience with independent living to better care for themselves and become part of community life.
2. Explain why persons with mental illness and their advocates have been more challenged to achieve parity in healthcare benefits and community services to meet their needs than other groups of persons with disabilities, such as children with development disabilities and their advocates.
3. Differentiate the types of intervention provided by an occupational therapy practitioner and a social worker on an assertive outreach team. Utilize an occupational therapy practice model or frame of reference to illustrate these differences and relate them to evaluation, intervention, and outcomes.
4. A unique feature of a clubhouse model of service for persons with mental illness is that all participants have equal value to the work of the clubhouse. What might this mean for occupational therapy evaluation and intervention?
5. As a consultant to a community program serving persons who are homeless, what specific interventions might you choose to provide? Can you produce evidence of the efficacy of these interventions? Propose a study that might help demonstrate the efficacy of specific occupational therapy interventions to reduce costs of maintaining people in a state of homelessness.

REFERENCES

Cottrell, R.P.F. (2007). The new freedom initiative-transferring mental health care: Will occupational therapy be at the table? *Occupational Therapy in Mental Health*, *23* (2) 1–25.

Darwish, A., Salmon, G., Ahuja, A. & Steed, L. (2006). The community intensive therapy team: Development and philosophy of a new service. *Clinical Child Psychology & Psychiatry, 11* (4), 591–605.

Eklund, M. (2006). Occupational factors and characteristics of social networks in people with persistent mental illness. *American Journal of Occupational Therapy, 60* (5) 587–594.

Eklund, M. (2007). Perceived control: How is it related to daily occupation in patients with mental illness living in the community? *American Journal of Occupational Therapy, 61* (5) 535–542.

Fisher, G.S. & Hotchkiss, A. (2008). A model of occupational empowerment for marginalized populations in community environments. *Occupational Therapy in Health Care, 22* (1) 55–71.

Gewurtz, R., Krupa, T., Eastabrook, S. & Horgan, S. (2004). Prevalence and characteristics of parenting among people served in assertive community treatment. *Psychiatric Rehabilitation Journal, 28* (1) 63–65.

Hafez, A. (2000). Case management practice. *The American Journal of Occupational Therapy, 54* (5) 114–115.

Herzberg, G. & Finlayson, M. (2001). Development of occupational therapy in a homeless shelter. *Occupational Therapy in Health Care, 13*, 133–148.

Hogan, M. (2003). The President's New Freedom Commission: Recommendations to transform mental health care in America. *Psychiatric Services, 54*, 1467–1474.

Killaspy, H., Johnson, S. & Bebbington, P. (2008). Developing mental health services in response to research evidence. *Epidemiologia E Psichiatria Sociale 17* (1) 47–56.

Meyer, P.S. & Morrissey, J.P. (2007). A comparison of assertive community treatment and intensive case management for patients in rural areas. *Psychiatric Services, 58* (1) 121–127.

Mitchell, H. & Jones, D. (2004) Homelessness: A review of the social policy background and the role of occupational therapy. *British Journal of Occupational Therapy, 67* (5) 315–319.

National Institutes of Mental Health (2008). Retrieved November 20, 2008 from *http://www.nimh.nih.gov/health/statistics/index.shtml*

New Freedom Commission on Mental Health (2003). *Achieving the promise: Transforming mental health care in America.* Washington, DC: Author.

Paterson, C. (2002). A short history of occupational therapy in psychiatry. In J. Creek (Ed.) *Occupational therapy in mental health* (pp. 3–14). London: Churchill Livingstone.

Peterson, M., Michael, W. & Armstrong, M. (2006). Homeward bound: Moving treatment from the institution to the community. *Administration and Policy in Mental Health, 33* (4) 508–511.

Russell, A. & Lloyd, C. (2004). Partnerships in mental health: Addressing barriers to social inclusion. *International Journal of Therapy and Rehabilitation, 11* (6) 267–274.

Scheinholz, M.K. (2001). Community-based mental health services. In M. Scaffa (Ed.) *Occupational therapy in community-based programs.* (pp. 291–312). Philadelphia, PA: F.A. Davis.

Schwartz, K.B. (2005). The history and philosophy of psychosocial occupational therapy. In E. Cara & A. McRae (Eds.) *Psychosocial occupational therapy: A clinical practice* (2nd ed., pp. 57–79). Clifton Park, NY: Thomson Delmar Learning.

Stein, F. & Cutler, S. (1998). *Psychosocial occupational therapy: A holistic approach.* San Diego, CA: Singular Publishing Group, Inc.

Tam, C. & Law, S. (2007). Best practices: A systematic approach to the management of patients who refuse medication in an assertive community treatment team setting. *Psychiatric Services, 58* (4) 457–459.

Tyrer, P., Balod, A., Germanavicus A., McDonald, A., Varadan, M. & Thomas, J. (2007). Perceptions of assertive community treatment in the UK and Lithuania. *International Journal of Social Psychiatry, 53* (6) 498–506.

Weissbrem-Padan, D., Vax, S., Naor, R., Sahar, N., Askayo, H., Tsabar, O., Austin, O., Soffer, A., Bouni, O. & Hadas-Lidor, N. (2006). Occupational therapy practice in Israel following community–based rehabilitation for people with psychiatric disability act 2000. *WFOT Bulletin, 53,* 36–43.

Section

III

DEVELOPING AND IMPLEMENTING YOUR OWN IDEAS FOR COMMUNITY PRACTICE

This section will guide you through conceptualizing to implementing the community practice you envision for yourself. It proposes a model of business development in which program planning, financing, marketing, and evaluation are integrated activities. If you have decided to practice in the community, your next consideration is whether to work in one of the practices already existing in your community or to develop and implement your own business. To start your own business you will need to assess your motives, skills, and abilities, as well as perform specific tasks to prepare yourself for success in community practice. This section assists you as you make the transition toward self-employment in the community. Many resources are available to help you along the way, and most of them can be found at a public library or online.

Envision a process of preplanning during which you identify your motives for starting a community practice and then explore the environment for opportunities and resources. The information gathered during this preplanning period should assure you that you can offer something valuable to others in your community and that your practice is likely to be economically feasible. After you have decided to develop a community practice, you begin a second phase of intensive planning that involves four main functions: business development, marketing, financing, and evaluation. By considering all simultaneously, you integrate the functions of business at

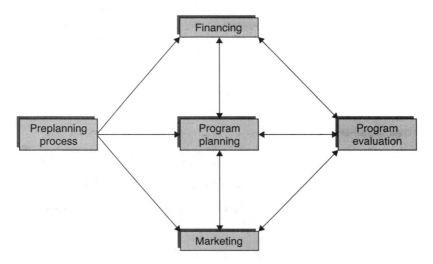

Figure SN3-1 Integrating business functions provides valuable feedback to community practitioners in a changing environment

the outset so that any activity you undertake supports the other functions. Although each of these functions is explained in detail—along with resources that will help you plan and implement your new community practice—each function is also discussed in relationship to the others.

The diagram above illustrates how each function relates to and impacts decision making for the others. First, the preplanning process of gathering data and reflecting on your own assets ends in a decision of whether or not you should move forward and develop your business. Preplanning contributes information that will be used as you develop your programming, marketing, and financing. The business development period will likely be the most challenging time of starting your practice because it requires many decisions that will influence the structure and success of your practice. These decisions will impact your marketing plans as well as determine how you will finance your community practice. I propose that you integrate the process of evaluation into developing your services and planning your financing and marketing. By integrating all these activities, you will likely build in mechanisms that can provide continuous feedback, allowing you to make decisions and respond to a changing environment as well as anticipated or unanticipated outcomes.

Chapter 7

Preplanning For Community Practice Development

- Analyze your motivation for developing a community practice.
- Explore the potential needs in your community for your services.
- Verify that your idea is financially feasible.

INTRODUCTION

Working in the community may not be for everyone, but there are different options for practice. You may choose to work in one of the many jobs that already exist in your community, such as in a school or as a home care therapist, or you may decide you want the challenge of developing an innovative practice. Although aspects of community practice may appear attractive compared to institutional practice, development of your own practice is a significant undertaking that requires motivation and skills. In order to determine if community practice will satisfy your work needs, you might consider systematically exploring your desire to become responsible for your own practice. As you take time to reflect upon your interests and attitudes, and review the stories from practice in earlier chapters, you may decide that the best place for you to practice occupational therapy is in an existing job in your community or that you will develop your own community practice. In addition to reviewing your comfort with the autonomy and flexibility required for some community practice, we will explore how collaboration with others is essential to starting and maintaining your practice. Collaboration involves identifying programs and people with whom occupational therapy practitioners can form synergistic relationships to improve life in our communities for persons with and without disabilities.

Scanning the environment is a preliminary task to development of your community practice. Before moving ahead with plans for independent practice, you will want to determine that a need exists in your community that you can satisfy with occupational therapy services and that there are enough potential clients to support your work. Just as you screen clients to determine whether occupational therapy would be beneficial, scanning the environment is a necessary precursor to further evaluating and developing your community practice.

SKILLS AND ATTITUDES TO CONSIDER BEFORE DEVELOPING A COMMUNITY PRACTICE

Flexibility

Community practice can be a grand adventure—an ideal opportunity to create your own practice, be your own manager, and perhaps even earn a substantial livelihood. Before making the decision to develop your own practice, however, you must assess your work habits and preferences. The opportunity to allow more flexibility in work hours is the impetus for some people to start their own businesses. Wanting to exercise more control over work life drives others to strike out on their own. If you prefer external structure to organize your work, having to develop and provide your own structure may be uncomfortable. Exceptional time management and organizational skills are important for success in private practice; you will need to be accountable to payers, clients, regulators, and any employees you may have. At the same time, it is important to remain flexible and recognize that you will not always be able to control all aspects of your work environment, even if it is your own business.

When things go wrong, and they sometimes do, you will need to adapt to the situation and keep your practice functioning to meet clients' needs. As you consider entering community practice, you will want to examine your own attitudes toward structure, both internal and external. You will need to be flexible regarding service delivery and not be frustrated with changes beyond your control, even when they may affect your financial outcomes. Your income is affected when clients cancel their appointments, or are not home when you arrive for a scheduled visit. Other times it may seem as though there are too many clients to be seen in one regular work day. In home-based practice, for example, clients consider their care provider to be someone they trust and can contact whenever they have concerns about their health condition. Health care is a service industry and you must examine your feelings about being responsive to meet the needs of your clients outside of usual work hours.

People who operate their own businesses know that to be successful they need to meet clients' needs and exceed expectations for service (Stephenson & Mintzer, 2008). You will need to be flexible in order to fit unscheduled phone calls, or even a visit, into a work day that may already be fully scheduled. Depending on your perspective, this can be viewed as either a frustration or an achievable challenge. A therapist's attitude toward unpredictable events will determine success in community practice. An occupational therapy practitioner in community practice maintains a flexible schedule while understanding that any adjustments to it cannot be attributed to any one person or event, but rather are the nature of the work she has chosen. Clients prefer their providers to be positive, client centered, and reliable. The success of any private practice depends on satisfied clients. It would therefore be an advantage to be naturally easy-going and able to manage your own stress in a healthy way.

Accepting Differences in Others

If you decide to provide home services, flexibility and acceptance of others' lifestyles are required because you may work in environments that seem disorganized or dirty. Seeing a young child for therapy in his home may require collaborating in an environment where sisters or brothers are present, engaged in active play, and contributing considerable noise and distraction to therapy. This is the child's usual environment, however, and one in which the therapist must either adapt or effect change in order to be successful. Visiting an adult client at home may include the presence of family members, friends, and sometimes pets. Dogs bark, and occasionally growl; cats brush back and forth against your legs, covering them with fur, and family and friends carry on with their conversations and activities in the midst of therapy. Although the activity and noise of the people and pets in the client's environment may seem chaotic or unpleasant to you, it is the atmosphere in which your client must function every day. You will need to remain focused on your work with your client despite these distractions. This does not mean that family members and friends should be ignored. Their involvement with the client is part of home living, so developing strategies to engage them with the client may be an important aspect of therapy. On the other hand, it is not unreasonable to ask that pets be secured during your visit if they are threatening or provoke allergies. In community work, you must be assertive when necessary while also welcoming opportunities to involve family or friends in therapy sessions. People who are significant to the client can become an important adjunct to your treatment. They can learn more about the abilities of the client and can help a client function at his highest level.

Home is the domain of the client who lives there and reflects the client's preference for order and cleanliness. Working in homes that are not cleaned to your standards may prove a challenge. Some client homes have dirty floors, bathrooms, and kitchens, as well as disorder throughout. Unless these living conditions contribute to a client's distress, however, they are a client's choice and adapting to accommodate these environments is part of home practice. A home based therapist recently told me about visiting a client with an extensive firearms collection, which he proudly displayed in his home. The therapist was advised before his first visit that the firearms were in the home, since this situation resulted in other therapists refusing to visit this client. While the guns were not threatening to this therapist, and in fact provided a topic for discussion during treatment, another therapist perceived their presence as a threat. Clients or their family members may practice a variety of different customs, such as removing shoes when entering the home. Adapting to these customs will facilitate a better therapeutic relationship and contribute to better service outcomes.

Managing Time

Working in the community requires good time management skills. Establishing priorities and having an awareness of time are essential. There are different methods of time management, but most begin with first identifying daily, weekly, and monthly activities essential to maintaining your practice, and developing a schedule for yourself that contains these and any other activities you would like to do. Each week must be carefully planned to include time for visits, travel from one client to the next if necessary, meetings, treatment planning, documentation, billing, and other financial and legal obligations of practice. In the absence of externally regulated work hours, such as those specified by an employer, you may be tempted to spend time on non-work activities during the day. People who have been unsuccessful in a job that required working from home often cite the frustration of trying to multitask home and work activities. While having flexibility in work hours may be an advantage of community practice, successfully integrating non-work activities with work activities remains your responsibility and requires prioritizing everything important to your personal and work objectives. There are tools for accomplishing this, such as day planners and electronic organizers, and strategies such as prioritizing tasks and organizing specific blocks of time for them (Stephenson & Mintzer, 2008). The saying "time is money" has real consequences in any community practice where your income depends directly on producing billable hours.

Autonomy in Practice

A desire for autonomy may be what attracts you to community practice. You believe that you have good time management skills and can tolerate lifestyles that differ from your own. You want to have control of your work life and not be managed by someone else. Autonomy, however, also means forfeiting opportunities to socialize with other therapists as part of each work day. This can be a stumbling block to practice as an independent service provider if you enjoy sharing ideas and responsibilities with peers on a daily basis. On the other hand, if you enjoy challenges and problem solving, independent practice may be ideal for you. Autonomy doesn't imply a reluctance to work with others, but simply a confidence in your ability to work independently. When necessary, you will be able to reach out for assistance to a support network of other therapists who have chosen to work in the community.

The ability to locate or form a network of therapists engaged in similar occupational therapy practice may be a high priority, especially when you are beginning a new community practice. Some therapists engaged in independent practice form groups that meet regularly to discuss common issues and participate in continuing education programs to upgrade their skills and knowledge. An available network of other therapists willing to listen and offer support provides options for discussing the challenges that arise regularly in any practice. The internet provides opportunities to seek out colleagues, both near and far, who share your interests in practice. It also provides opportunities to consult with experts, and to connect with colleagues at a time convenient to you. Ladies Who Launch is an organization that provides networking opportunities to women who either are considering starting a business or who own small businesses.

MOTIVATION FOR COMMUNITY PRACTICE

Establishment of a community practice will require a lot of hard work and may not happen quickly. You will want to be certain that your motivation to undertake this endeavor is enough to sustain you through the process. Listing your reasons for wanting to develop your own practice is helpful.

Barringer and Ireland (2008) identify triggers to starting a new business, such as having a great idea, experiencing a change in family status, undergoing a change in financial status, reaching a developmental or age milestone, or retiring. Acting on any of these triggers must be accompanied by recognizing and nurturing any personal characteristics and strengths that would predict business success, including persistence, patience, self-confidence, commitment, resilience, and energy (Marks, 2006).

The Great Idea

Most people who go into business for themselves move into an area in which they already have some expertise. You may know that your clinical skills are highly desired in your community and that you would have many clients if you were to have your own practice. If you have been working with children over a long period of time, you are likely to have identified some services for these children that may be missing in your community. For example, a therapist who had been working with children in an early intervention program continued to see some of her clients past the age when they could receive home based government reimbursed services and was instead reimbursed through private payment by their parents or their insurance. As these children reached school age, several parents reported that although their children received therapy in school, they struggled academically. In addition, no tutoring services were available in the community for children with disabilities. This therapist's idea to develop a program to offer tutoring for these children emerged from a need identified by parents. If you have been working with older adults you may have some idea of services they would like to receive in their home or community. Whatever your areas of practice or expertise, you probably have some ideas that could be developed into a community practice.

Working for Yourself

Probably the main motivator for people to start a business is the idea that working for themselves has significantly greater appeal than working for someone else (Peters, 2005). There is no doubt that health care has changed and continues to change in ways that challenge those who work in institutions. The economics of health care dictate practice. Amount of payment for services, what can be treated, length and frequency of treatment, and in some cases even the treatment protocol, are all dictated by economic considerations. Productivity requirements have increased in response to these challenges. A therapist has little time to establish a relationship with her clients before they have gone home or to another treatment facility. Documentation requirements are significant and have little appeal for some therapy practitioners. These demands for time and energy, in the absence of opportunity to establish a relationship with clients, have been a catalyst for many therapists to leave institutional settings for a practice where they can set their own tempo for work that is more satisfying.

To work with the type of clients you prefer, perhaps for fewer or more rewarding hours, without external productivity demands, and in some cases unappreciative administrators, are all reasons why you might choose to develop a community practice. As economic pressures mount, some therapists working in institutional environments may find their jobs eliminated. When this phenomenon occurred in the late 1990s, therapists reluctant to find another job working for an institution decided community practice would be preferable as it would let them have more control over their work life.

Risk Taking: Making the Leap

If you discover that you have ideas on developing your own practice and would like to work for yourself, you still have to assess how comfortable you are taking risks. Starting your own business has associated risks, although not everyone becoming an independent practitioner assumes the same ones. One major risk may be loss of income and benefits that accrue from working for an established employer. If you have a life partner who is employed and can cover your health insurance needs, you may be able to take part-time work that gives you sufficient income while you develop a community practice. You may also have savings that allow you the freedom to choose your work.

For most people, the risk that creates the greatest fear is losing money invested in starting a small business (Stephenson & Mintzer, 2008). If economic insecurity is something you think you cannot tolerate, you might put this into perspective by considering that the cost to start most small businesses is fairly small; the average cost is $10,000, most of which comes from personal savings (Wells Fargo Bank, 2006). If you do not take the risk, however, you also cannot know the rewards that come with implementing your great ideas, and the satisfaction that comes from being successful in your own business (Solie-Johnson, 2005). Barrington and Ireland (2008) state that business owners are moderate risk takers; they take calculated risks by being well-informed of the opportunities in the environment that predict success and by getting advice from experts.

COMMUNITY COLLABORATION PROVIDES OPPORTUNITIES FOR PRACTICE

Community practice requires knowledge of existing programs and services and provides opportunities to enhance the quality of life for all residents, including your potential clients. By reaching out and collaborating with existing services, you may provide new or enhanced opportunities for persons with differing abilities to participate in community life. Institutional practice calls for teamwork among healthcare professionals, but in community practice your team will consist largely of persons who are not healthcare practitioners. One of the objectives of community treatment is to integrate clients into their own communities. Your efforts to collaborate and make services accessible to all will strengthen your community (Baum, 2007).

The occupational therapy practice framework identifies the importance of participation in community life (AOTA, 2008). Whether you work with persons with physical or mental disabilities, all your clients—and all citizens of your community—share the right to participate in work, school, home, and community life. To be effective in providing activities and advocating for the participation of persons with disabilities, you must be aware of the types of activities people in your community enjoy doing, and understand that these activities reflect the culture within which your client lives. Depending on your location, people in your community may enjoy skiing, bowling, beachcombing, or visiting museums. Most likely your clients would like to participate in the same activities enjoyed by others in the community. Begin exploring all the different types of activities offered publicly in your community. Doing so will help you recommend activities to your clients, knowing they would be welcomed as a community participant.

When searching out leisure activities, visit local parks and look for play equipment, walking trails, and swimming pools. Your local parks department may offer organized sports and recreation opportunities that would welcome people with disabilities. Some communities offer swimming programs for persons with physical disabilities where help is available with dressing as well as entering and exiting the pool. You may encounter exercise programs that meet in the community and can accommodate individuals with differing physical abilities. Art, history, or other lectures offered at area arts centers or libraries may be of interest and accessible to your clients. Classes that develop artistic expression, such as painting or ceramics, may be available to all interested community residents. Some communities offer programs such as movies or cooking groups for persons with special needs. Groups of mothers with young children may meet to support each other while enjoying social or recreational activities. Courses offered to teach new skills or develop hobbies are opportunities for persons with disabilities to learn and socialize. Where these programs are offered, you can suggest them to your clients. Where they do not yet exist, there may be opportunity for you to develop leisure activities to accommodate people with special needs.

As a community based occupational therapy practitioner, your search for activities of all types begins with contacting directors of community programs or by visiting the activity itself to see if it accommodates your client's needs of cost, accessibility, and inclusion with or without support. Your initial contact with a program provider begins a collaborative process linking community resources to persons with differing abilities. In a convenient place, keep some sort of file or binder that contains all relevant information about community activities, such as meeting times, costs, name of a contact person, phone number, and address. You can access these materials to plan a client's community integration.

Most communities organize special programs for their elders that include social activities or meals. Some programs offer day care or respite care for families who are caring for an elder with special needs in their home. Contacting these programs, and establishing rapport with their staff, will assist you in offering community resources to families caring for elders, and help you locate opportunities for elders to engage in meaningful social and task activities.

Most people desire to work, even if they are unable to hold a paying job. Work gives meaning to the lives of many of our clients. Volunteers are needed by community agencies and programs. Identifying volunteer opportunities and the type of work needed can help match a client who wants to work with an agency needing volunteer help. Establishing a collaborative relationship with organizers in agencies welcoming volunteers may facilitate accommodations for persons with different physical or cognitive abilities, and further extends the reach of occupational therapy into the community.

Children with disabilities need activities that meet their needs to learn, be creative, and socialize. Children who attend either special or regular schools may not have equal access to the sports and arts programs enjoyed by non-disabled children. If the organization Special Olympics is active and available in your community, consider contacting it and offering to volunteer with its sports programs. You may benefit by getting acquainted with participants and families who may need your services. This can provide an important networking opportunity as you develop your community practice.

A childhood opportunity to experiment with the arts may lead to a lifelong love of music, dance, or other arts. Collaboration between an occupational therapy practitioner and a dance school could result in movement classes for children with special needs. Music can also be adapted for different abilities. Inclusion into these arts programs enhances quality of life for children as it integrates them with their non-disabled peers. It also rewards the occupational therapy practitioner who has facilitated these opportunities, as he observes the child with a disability become part of the community.

Camping is a special experience of youth. It often is the child's first experience away from his parents in which special friendships develop with peers. It is a time of learning skills of independence, sports, and recreation, and it is even fun. Many adults have fond memories of songs they learned at camp, along with special camp food and activities.

Camping is another area of community practice where occupational therapy practitioners may collaborate with others within the community to provide an experience for children or adults with disabilities. Camps for non-disabled children and young adults may either include young people with special needs, or set aside special times when staff can accommodate healthcare providers offering camping opportunities for children and adults with special needs. Such special camping experiences will most often include volunteer healthcare providers such as occupational and physical therapists, nurses, and students to assist the campers. If not yet offered in your community, camping may provide an excellent opportunity for you to collaborate with other healthcare professionals and develop a rewarding camping experience with an organization that already operates camps for non-disabled children. Planning or adapting camping activities for children with special needs, or arranging for volunteers to assist children and young adults with disabilities while they attend a community camp, would enhance the regular camping program. A camping program for children or adults with disabilities provides an additional benefit by allowing their parents or other caregivers to have a respite from the responsibilities of providing care.

An occupational therapy practitioner who collaborates with community programs and agencies will be educating others in her community about the need for all people to have meaningful occupations, including leisure, work, and social opportunities. She will also help these programs and agencies to adapt their activities to accommodate people with special needs. Occupational therapy becomes a method of promoting social justice by providing the education and means to integrate people with disabilities into community activities. Hinojosa (2007) states that therapists must work in partnership with others to integrate clients in activities that give their lives meaning.

SCANNING THE ENVIRONMENT

Scanning the environment is a precursor to further developing your community practice. Gathering and analyzing information about your community, its residents, and their needs, along with identifying potential clients for services you would like to offer, is necessary before you begin to develop a business plan. Preliminary data will be used to make decisions about the type of practice that would be welcomed in your community, and will minimize your risk of developing an unsuccessful practice.

What is Needed by Your Community?

As you begin scanning your environment, ask yourself if a need exists in your community for your great idea for practice. If you are new to the community, you will need to learn as much as possible about its residents, their work, and their leisure activities. Most people, however, develop businesses in communities where they have resided for some time and are familiar with local people and customs. While living and working in a community, you may identify a service needed by residents that either does not currently exist or that you could provide more effectively. The question you need to find an answer to in your environmental scan is: "Is there a sufficient need for this service to support my desire to provide it?" You may already know the answer to this question if you have identified enough potential clients from among the people with whom you currently work.

It is likely, however, that you will need to collect additional information about a need for services. You can talk to people who may have access to future clients, such as physicians or managers of other community services, or to support groups of people who care for your potential clients. Explain who you are, what you can provide, and any special expertise you may have. Ask what types of services are needed in your community and whether clients would be willing to pay for them. You may want to explore how potential clients would pay for services. Would they expect third-party payment or would they pay privately? How much would the services be worth to them? Talking to as many different people as possible during this exploratory stage of practice development will help you better understand the community and its needs. At this stage of scanning the environment, a reference librarian in your community is a good resource. She can lead you to demographic information on your community and offer her insights as a fellow resident (Barringer & Ireland, 2008).

Are There Competitors?

Services similar or identical to the services you would like to offer may already exist in your community. You will need to learn about these services, their providers, locations, and hours of operation to develop a practice that will be competitive or complementary. You can find community practices identical or similar to the type you are considering by accessing the internet to locate directories of providers in your state. Medline Plus, a service of the National Library of Medicine and the National Institutes of Health, provides lists of services and providers by state and zip code or county. To learn more about how similar practices operate, you can read articles in magazines geared toward small businesses such as *Entrepreneur, Small Business, Inc,* or *Fortune* to better understand challenges and success strategies to build your confidence as you plan your practice. You can access census data about the population of your community including ages of residents, their disability status, their income and education levels, and where they live and work through the United States Census Bureau. The census data identifies prevalence of disabilities by type and age group. Comparing prevalence of persons with disabilities with availability of already existing services can reveal an unmet need within your community that you can address with your community practice.

To help you make decisions about services you would offer clients, visit practices that might be your competition and talk to the people who are currently providing services to the population you would like to serve. You want to know if they have a waiting list, or if clients want any services that competitors are unable or unwilling to offer. The information you are seeking in talking to competitors is:

- What specific services do clients want or need?
- How many potential clients can you identify who would use your service if it were offered today?
- If you offered the service, where would your prospective clients prefer to have it provided? Would they want home services or a certain community location?
- What would your potential clients be willing to pay for your services?

The answers to these questions help you determine if there is sufficient demand in your community to develop your practice. The information may also help you to modify your ideas to better meet needs and increase your potential for success.

Financing Options to Consider

Money is a factor that must be considered as a precursor to business development. Solie-Johnson (2005) suggests that you look to others to finance your business in order to share the risk. Another view is that you depend on your own resources to start your practice in order to maintain tighter control of your business (Barringer & Ireland, 2008). You will need some money to get your practice started, however, and will want to identify potential sources for financing, such as your own savings, money from family or friends willing to invest in your practice, or a loan from an outside source. The current economic climate is challenging for individuals who would like to start a small business; some usual sources of financing are unwilling to risk investing in new ventures. In the chapter about financing your practice, we will discuss some possible external funding options and methods of locating loans. Local banks are a possible source of startup funds; you can inquire whether a bank you are familiar with would provide a loan to start a private practice. You can also peruse the Web site of the Small Business Development Center of the Small Business Administration (SBA) for loan information. The SBA does not lend money, but it can assist you in identifying whether a loan is possible, where you might obtain the loan, and how to package a loan application (Solie-Johnson, 2005). You will not be in a position to actually negotiate a loan until you are further along in the development of your community practice, but at least knowing there is potential funding is important before proceeding with the next phase of development.

Having scanned the environment and determined that potential for successful development of your practice exists, you ask yourself: "Can I support myself doing this?" or "Can I earn what I believe my skills and knowledge are worth doing this?" If the answer to either of these questions is yes, you will proceed with the next steps in developing your practice knowing that the money you earn will be yours; you do not have to contribute to the salary of an administrator or add value to the work of an institution whose beliefs may or may not agree with your own. You can move forward knowing that you provide something that reflects your values and talents, and that it will be welcomed by your community.

CHAPTER SUMMARY

This chapter describes the preplanning process that you should undertake before making a decision to develop a community practice. You need to be sure you are flexible and resourceful, manage time well, and like to be autonomous and responsible for your own work. You have ideas you believe in, accept the challenge of making money, will work hard to achieve you dreams, and view risks as manageable. In addition to your personal reflections, you will have surveyed the environment and determined that there are people who would like to have and will pay for your services. You have begun identifying potential sources of funding to get your practice started. When this pre-planning process is completed, you will have the information necessary to decide whether to go forward with developing your own business, locate employment in an already established community practice that offers some of the benefits of having your own business, or remain with a familiar institutional practice.

LEARNING ACTIVITIES

The activities for this chapter are designed to assist you in assessing your skills, abilities, interests, and needs as well as the needs of your community for your services. Outcomes of these activities that will be useful as you move through planning and implementing your community practice and will become part of any funding request include:

- A brief resume stating your qualifications to develop and implement a community practice
- Statement of purpose for your proposed program

1. Becoming aware of your skills, knowledge, and any experiences that will contribute to your success in community practice will also contribute to your confidence to proceed.

   What idea have you formulated for your community practice? Compare your own professional skills, knowledge, and experiences with those needed to deliver these services. Include years of practice, specialized practice, certifications, or additional education.

   What experience do you have with working independently, collaborating with others in your community, assertiveness, multitasking, and money management? Identify each area and list the experience and its outcome. Relevant experiences may not necessarily be associated with your work as an occupational therapy practitioner.

Utilizing your list of attributes, prepare a short resume that describes you as a person who has achieved success, been responsible, and experienced increased independence in work.

2. Write a description of your community including population density, housing type, work performed by residents, major employers, education, preferred leisure activities, socioeconomic status, race, culture, and family structure.
3. What services are available for children or adults with disabilities to participate in work, education, and leisure activities in your community? Identify any programs or services that are intended solely for persons with disabilities and any programs that include persons with disabilities. Are there desired activities or services identified by members of the community that you would like to provide?
4. Prepare a statement explaining what people in your community want or need that you will provide in your community practice.

REFERENCES

American Occupational Therapy Association (2008). Occupational therapy practice framework: Domain and Process (2nd ed). *The American Journal of Occupational Therapy, 62* (6) 625–683.

Barringer, B.R. & Ireland, R.D. (2008). *What's stopping you? Shattering the 9 most common myths keeping you form starting your own business.* Upper Saddle River, NJ: Pearson Education Inc.

Baum, C. (2007). Farewell presidential address, 2007: Achieving our potential. *The American Journal of Occupational Therapy, 61* (6) 615–621.

Hinojosa, J. (2007). Eleanor Clarke Slagle Lecture: Becoming innovators in an era of hyperchange. *The American Journal of Occupational Therapy, 61* (6) 629–637.

Marks, G. (2006). *Small Business Book of Lists.* Avon, MA: Adams Media.

Peters, T. (2005). *Re-imagine! Business excellence in a disruptive age.* London: Dorling Kindersley.

Solie-Johnson, K. (2005). *How to set up your own small business: Volume 1.* Minneapolis, MN: American Institute of Small Businesses.

Stephenson, J. & Mintzer, R. (2008). *Ultimate homebased business handbook* (2nd ed). Madison, WI: CWL Publishing Enterprises, Inc./ Entrepreneur Press.

Wells Fargo/ Small Business Index (2006). *How much money does it take to start a small business?* San Francisco, CA: Wells Fargo Bank.

ELECTRONIC SOURCES

Health information and rehabilitation service directories:
Medlineplus. Retrieved December 9, 2008 from http://www.nlm.nih.gov/medlineplus/rehabilitation

Census data of population trends for your community:
  U.S. Census Bureau. Retrieved December 9, 2008 from
  http://factfinder.census.gov
  http://www.fedstats.gov

Ladies Who Launch provides networking opportunities to women starting
or owning a business:
  (http://www.ladieswholaunch.com). Accessed on February 2, 2009.

Small Business Development Center, Small Business Administration:
  (http://www.sba.gov/sbdc). Accessed on February 2, 2009.

Chapter 8

Developing Your Practice

LEARNING OBJECTIVES

- Integrate professional skills and knowledge with practical considerations of developing a practice.
- Explain regulations that affect a practice.
- Evaluate the value of working with other professionals as you move forward in developing your practice.

INTRODUCTION

This chapter covers the basic decisions you will need to make as you get ready to establish a new occupational therapy practice in the community. You will need to be very specific about what you plan to offer in your practice. You will base your decisions on preliminary planning including your scan of the environment and an assessment of your existing skills and knowledge. You must decide whether to establish a solo practice, partnership, or group practice. Federal, state, and professional regulations will affect how you practice in your community. Explore opportunities to work with legal and accounting professionals as you plan your practice. Identify possible funding resources that will accommodate your practice plans and lead you to success. Begin developing a plan to seek financing. Suggestions for helpful resources to reach each decision will be found in this chapter and the following chapters about financing and marketing your program, both of which are also necessary to developing and implementing a business plan.

DECISIONS REGARDING THE SERVICE YOU WILL OFFER

Clinical Perspective: Evidence-Based Practice

At the conclusion of the pre-planning phase of developing your practice, you will have determined that your education and experience have provided you with the skills and knowledge to address the specific needs you have identified in your community. Before developing a business plan outlining the services you will provide, take time to investigate the literature to identify evidence that you will be offering the best possible clinical services to your clients. One of the biggest challenges to therapists using evidence-based practice is lack of time to complete a literature review (Corcoran, 2006; McKenna et al., 2005). This is an inadequate excuse for anyone considering building a community practice, because time spent identifying best practice is an investment in your outcomes. Bailey, Bornstein, and Ryan (2007) write that therapists building a practice must find and use examples of best practice as they plan how they will provide client care. Building your practice on the best available evidence may help you differentiate your practice from competitors in your community.

More recent graduates will have experience finding and evaluating evidence related to clinical practice. If the process of evidence-based practice is new to you, there are resources to help you get started. Law and MacDermid (2008) describe how to find, assess, and utilize literature in client centered practice. Addy (2006) demonstrates the application of evidence-based practice in physical rehabilitation through case studies, while Long and Cronin-Davis (2006) describe its application for mental health clients. Additional examples of evidence relevant to practice with specific populations can be found in professional journals.

Online occupational therapy resources are available to search multiple relevant databases: Two resources are the Evidence-Based Practice Resource Directory, administered by the American Occupational Therapy Association, and the international resource OTseeker (Bennett, Hoffman, McCluskey, McKenna, Strong & Tooth, 2003). To get started with either resource, you will need to identify the population and types of interventions you are considering for your practice, such as therapy for children with autism or driving assessments for older adults. The resulting list of articles can be winnowed down to those most relevant to your needs by reading the article abstract to determine type of study and outcomes. Read the articles you select as most relevant to your practice thoroughly. Make copies of articles that will contribute most to your decisions about interventions and discuss them with others who have knowledge of your proposed practice area.

Use the outcomes of these discussions to make decisions regarding what services you will offer. Identifying others with clinical expertise in your area of interest not only gives you someone with whom to discuss the evidence you have found, it also may provide you with someone who can serve as your mentor or consultant as you continue to develop your practice. Having someone with experience to talk with as you proceed will be very helpful, especially when decisions must be made or when things do not go exactly as planned.

Polatajko and Craik (2006) write that not all of the information needed to develop best practice is located in occupational therapy journals. They identify a large body of resources generated by other disciplines but applicable to occupational therapy. This may be especially relevant if you are developing a community practice that will utilize your professional skills and knowledge but will include aspects that may be new to occupational therapy. There may be other occupational therapy practitioners providing the type of practice you plan to offer, but no research or outcome studies published in occupational therapy journals. Apply the research published in other disciplines by reflecting thoughtfully on articles related to your proposed practice or by discussing the results with a peer familiar with your intended practice area (Polatajko & Craik, 2006). Bailey, Bornstein, and Ryan (2007) identify free or low-cost databases that will take you outside the occupational therapy literature. These include CINAHL, a database that searches allied health and nursing literature at a minimal cost. Access to a university library in your area would be optimal because literature searches may be free or low cost, but many public libraries can also help you search for evidence to support efficacy of interventions on which you plan to build your practice.

Knowing the Needs of Your Community

During your pre-planning process, you will have already surveyed your community to determine whether there is a need for services you would like to provide. Additional exploration of existing community resources needs to be done followed by an analysis to determine how your services might differ from those already available. If you did not meet with potential competitors as you scanned your environment, make appointments to speak with the practice managers of competitors. Gather any brochures or other promotional information related to the practices and visit their Web sites. If a potential competitor has more clients than it can serve, it may be willing to share them with you, especially if your services are directed toward specific populations or interventions they prefer to avoid. Do not be discouraged if you get a negative response from a potential competitor. If you can find no local practice similar to the one you propose, go online and see if you can locate a practice similar to yours in a different city or state. Arrange to speak with its manager.

As you collect information about community needs, you may discover that needs exist that you had not anticipated, and decide to include those in your practice. A Strengths, Weaknesses, Opportunities, and Threats (SWOT) analysis may help you identify how clients might view your services compared to those of competitors (Stephenson & Mintzer, 2008). Make a SWOT analysis for your practice and for the competition and compare the results. Strengths and weaknesses may include specialized skills, years of experience, certifications, equipment, referral sources, or financial assets of your practice compared to competitors. Opportunities arise from identifying trends such as rapidly aging populations, or identifying your strengths and utilizing them to meet a need that may not be met by a competitor. Threats are negative situations in the environment that can adversely affect the success of your practice, such as healthcare reimbursement practices or changes in government regulations that affect your practice. Initial SWOT analyses can assist you in deciding what to offer your community when you begin your practice, but as your practice matures, repeating this process can provide directions for expansion of services and ideas for continued business success.

Clients' preferences for accessing your services may be important to your success. Think about the hours and days of the week that are convenient for clients and make sure these are times you are able or willing to work. Services for retired adults are best offered during the day, Monday through Friday. In addition to having retired form paid employment, these aging adults are sometimes reluctant to go out after dark, and also may have many weekend activities planned. If you want to work with school-age children, however, you will need to consider working during after-school hours or on weekends to accommodate their availability. Most employed adults' work hours prevent them from being available for outside activities on weekdays until about 6 p.m. or later in the evening. An in-depth exploration of these considerations will contribute to your plans for marketing your practice, and may suggest you modify originally planned work hours to capture those clients looking for convenience as well as quality services. At this stage of developing your practice plan, information generated from the environment about unmet needs of individuals or groups, underserved populations, and preferences for time and location of service will assist you in your decision making process.

IMAGINE BEYOND THE USUAL: DEVELOP A BUSINESS PLAN

Having collected information about best practice and community opportunities, you will now begin to develop your practice plan. Your practice is a small business and you can follow procedures described in books written for small business entrepreneurs. The American Institute of Small Business publishes a step-by-step guide with many useful references (Solie-Johnson, 2005). Another helpful book that can be found at libraries or bookstores is *The Small Business Start-Up Kit*, which is a legal guide to establishing a business. This book identifies online resources and provides—both in the book as well as on an accompanying CD—copies of forms you will need to file to comply with federal and state regulations (Pakroo, 2008). The U.S. Chamber of Commerce has a Web site that includes a library of resources including how to start a business, develop a business plan, get financing, market your business, and manage finances and taxes. The Small Business Development Center offers free online training through self-paced video courses that include templates for developing a business plan. SCORE, a free nonprofit organization of retired executives, provides counseling and mentoring to entrepreneurs and maintains a Web site that offers templates to prepare a business plan, podcasts, and video instruction.

Mission Statement

Developing a business plan begins with creating a mission statement that is used to guide daily and future practice activities. The statement includes what the practice does, for whom, and in what context (Kotler, Hayes & Bloom, 2002). Mission statements are short and best kept to two or three sentences, but one sentence may be adequate to identify your practice's reason for existence. As you develop your mission statement, think about people you want to help, what they need, and how you can address those needs. Although you want to be expansive regarding what purpose your practice serves, be realistic about commitments you can make given the resources that you will have available, such as business loans and clients' abilities to pay for your service. If you are going to be a solo practitioner, you may also have limited time, human resources, space, and equipment to provide services to meet a wide array of demands. Write your statement and then think about what you have written. If your expectations are reasonable, continue to edit your statement so that your mission makes sense to others. The mission statement that you develop is included in your business plan along with your marketing literature when you approach anyone who might finance your practice. Make the statement clear, complete, and attractive to readers.

Describe Your Services

Your business plan continues by defining your potential clients' needs and what is currently available to meet those needs. Describe your potential clients including demographics of age, occupation, ability, socioeconomic status, or any other characteristics of clients that further defines who you will be serving through community practice.

Based on needs of clients, describe in detail the services you plan to offer and the expected outcomes of your efforts. Incorporate evidence of the efficacy of the specific evaluation and interventions you will offer clients. Your business plan must include what you plan to charge for each service. Methods for developing prices for your services are included in the chapter about financing your practice.

ON YOUR OWN OR WITH A PARTNER?

A business plan describes your practice's organization and management tasks. You may already have made the decision about whether you want to work alone or with others in your practice. Liability and tax implications for different types of practices will be described, but as you choose which seems to suit your needs best, you may want to obtain legal advice.

Advantages and Disadvantages of Solo Practice

If you have decided to work alone, you will own the assets of your practice and receive all profits. You will also assume complete responsibility for any liability and debt incurred by the practice (Marks, 2006). One advantage of starting practice as a sole practitioner is that you will not need to file papers to become a corporation; starting your practice will be fairly easy and you will not incur the cost of incorporation. As sole practitioner you will be able to transfer funds in and out of your business from your personal assets. You have total responsibility for your practice; you are the boss. You file federal and state tax returns using Internal Revenue Service (IRS) Schedule C to report your practice's profits and losses. An employer withholds money to cover taxes that must be paid to the government. As a sole proprietor, you will need to pay estimated federal and state taxes, including contributions to Social Security and Medicare, each quarter. Even if your business seems uncomplicated, it is advised that you consult with a tax expert to establish methods of tax payments (Pakroo, 2008). You can close a sole practitioner practice fairly easily, but it is difficult for you to expand this type of business to include others.

Working with a Partner

A second option for your practice is to join with one or more partners. Partners share ownership of the practice and should draw up a legal agreement about how decisions are made, profits are shared, disputes resolved, partners added or bought out, and steps taken to dissolve the partnership if necessary (Marks, 2006). There are three types of partnerships: general partnerships, limited partnerships, and limited liability partnerships. A general partnership brings two or more individuals together to form a practice with all partners personally liable for all business debts; each partner, however, has individual authority to enter into a contract. A limited partnership includes one general partner who controls business operations, and limited partners who have limited control over practice decisions in exchange for protection from personal liability (Pakroo, 2008). A limited liability partnership provides a business structure that shields partners' personal assets against liability and is preferred for professional services that may incur malpractice claims. This type of structure, permitted by most states, must be registered with your state. Before establishing a limited liability partnership, you will need to verify that according to your state regulations, your practice qualifies. The duration of a limited liability partnership is specified when it is registered with the state, but may be continued by vote of partners when registration expires. By going to the Web site for the Secretary of State for your state, you can find the information needed to determine if you can form this type of practice and also which forms you need to file with your state. This type of partnership provides the limited liability features of a corporation but retains tax efficiencies and management flexibility described for other partnerships (Marks, 2006). If you become a limited liability partnership, assets of the practice are distributed to its partners, who pay individual tax on this income. This is an easy partnership to establish with minimal cost for filing with your state.

Incorporation

Taxes and liabilities differ with more complex business structures. Consulting with an accountant or an attorney is advisable before establishing a corporation. Briefly, a corporation is a business chartered by the state and legally considered to be separate from its owners. A corporation is taxed, can be sued, and can enter into contractual agreements; its owners elect a board of directors to develop and assure compliance with its policies and decisions. When a member leaves, the corporation continues. A corporation is taxed differently than partnerships and requires separate tax filing. An S corporation enables its directors to treat earnings and profits as distributions and pass them directly to their personal tax returns. Corporations require a director and development of bylaws. (Pakroo, 2008). Practices that are state-incorporated must be renewed annually by filing the appropriate forms and paying the fee established by your state. You will need to register with your state if you are a partnership organization.

Choosing the best structure for your practice requires decisions about shared responsibility and tax liability. The various options available are best discussed in consultation with legal and accounting experts who can help you determine the best structure for your practice.

WILL YOU BE FOR PROFIT, NONPROFIT, OR COLLABORATE WITH A NONPROFIT ORGANIZATION?

Most community practices will be operated for profit. If, however, you want your business to be a nonprofit organization, there are specific procedures that you must undertake. You can register and incorporate your practice as a nonprofit organization with your state. This does not, however, give you status as a 501-(c)-(3) organization with the IRS, which provides tax advantages and is required for most grant awards. Describing the process of becoming a nonprofit organization is beyond the scope of this book. If you want to consider becoming a nonprofit organization, a very helpful book is *How to Form a Nonprofit Corporation,* which you can find at bookstores or your public library. This book will take you step-by-step through the process of developing a nonprofit organization and includes forms and sample documents required to apply to become a nonprofit organization (Mancuso, 2007). While there are tax advantages to forming a nonprofit 501-(c)-(3) organization, this is a complex and lengthy process and you will be unable to make decisions for the organization and simultaneously be paid by the organization. If you want to start a community practice and would like the benefit of applying for a grant, you could consider partnering with a nonprofit organization in your community with which you share interests. Your services would be an extension of the nonprofit organization, you would be compensated as an independent contractor, and you would build into any grant application or other agreement with the organization your salary, benefits, and other terms of employment. Such a mutually beneficial arrangement can allow you to share responsibility for the programs you develop with the organization, which as a result can better serve its own community purposes.

CHOOSING A NAME

Deciding on a name for your practice can be challenging, but perhaps you had a name in mind when you first began thinking about establishing a community practice. Consider choosing a name that reflects what you do, is easily remembered, and is not already used by another business. Although most small businesses use the name of the person starting the business, healthcare practices are more likely to have a name that reflects services offered so that potential clients searching for care have a logical point of reference. Including such terms as "rehabilitation" in combination with "kids," "driving," or "home," would attract people interested in your services. A short name is easier to remember than a long name. To avoid confusing potential clients, do not select a name that too closely resembles the name of another business in your community. Legal issues also can arise if the name you choose has already been legally protected by another business (Pakroo, 2008; Stephenson & Mintzer, 2008). If you plan to incorporate in your state, you will be unable to complete incorporation with a name already in use by another corporation in your state. To determine whether you will be able to use the name you have chosen, go to the Web site for your Secretary of State and search the database that lists all names of incorporated businesses. Additional legal complications can arise with names that have been claimed by others, such as names that have been trademarked (Pakroo, 2008). To see whether the name you want to use is protected by trademark or other protection, consult federal government business Web sites that will link you to databases of registered business names. If the name you would like to use for your practice is not listed as in use by another business in your state, and is not protected by federal trademark or copyright, you can select this name for your practice.

You likely will want to include the internet in your marketing practices, therefore it is desirable to use the same name chosen for your practice for your Web site. To see if this is possible, you will need to determine if the domain name you would like to use is already being used by someone else. Find out whether the domain name you want to use is available by searching online with an internet information center. If the name you want to use for your Web site is not already in use by another organization, you can register it. If it is already taken, you can experiment with other options that incorporate your practice name to see if they are available. With a little persistence, usually you can find a domain name that is close enough to your practice name that clients can find you on the Web.

IS THIS FEASIBLE? AM I READY TO TAKE THE RISK?

As you work though developing your business plan and selecting a name, take time to reflect on what you have accomplished. Make sure that you want to proceed and that you are willing to take necessary risks to succeed in your own community practice. The people who succeed as entrepreneurs have some things in common: they like to make money, have big dreams, are success oriented, work harder than most people, and are better than most others at what they do. They love a challenge, learn from mistakes, and maintain a high level of integrity in their work (Solie-Johnson, 2005). Peters (2005) makes a compelling argument for going forward with your plans when he says that if you have talent, use it and profit rather than let your efforts continue to support organizational management.

REGULATIONS OF PRACTICE

Your practice will be regulated by government and professional organizations. These regulations will vary depending on your state of residence. As you proceed with developing your practice, consult your state and local government, along with state and local chapters of professional organizations, for information on practice and business requirements.. A few general considerations, however, will be discussed here so that you can familiarize yourself with what you need to look for as you establish your community practice.

Professional Practice Guidelines

If your practice is going to be provided as a professional service, and especially if you intend to bill as a professional service, you will need to be in full compliance with your state practice act. You should print a copy of your state practice act from your state's professional regulations Web site. Review each section as you plan your practice to be certain you adhere to the provisions of practice regarding what you can and cannot do as a professional. You may need to modify your practice plan in response to regulations, but you must be in compliance or you will be subject to losing your credentials to practice. Occupational therapy services should also be consistent with the Occupational Therapy Practice Framework, 2nd edition (AOTA, 2008).

State Regulations

Every state has health and safety regulations that will apply to your practice. Your state Board of Health will oversee your compliance with these regulations through review of your records and on-site visits. Get a copy of the regulations that apply in your state, and as you set up your location, be sure that you are in compliance with fire safety, building codes, and infection control policies. Establishing procedures that follow federal and state guidelines for medical records is essential. This will involve purchasing secured storage for these documents, although you may want to consider purchasing a medical records management program that can in the future be linked to a national data system for medical records. Most likely you have worked in the past for an organization that has undergone reviews and on-site visits by regulators who assure safe and secure service delivery to the public. Use these past experiences to your benefit as your set up our own practice.

Tax Regulations

Your state will require that you register your business, unless you are a sole proprietor, in which case you must comply with general state and federal tax codes. If you have employees, you will need to register for an Employee Identification Number (EIN) from the Internal Revenue Service to report earnings of your employees. This process can be completed by going to the IRS Web site and downloading Form SS-4 or filing the form online. Once the form is received by the IRS, they will send you your EIN and additional information about being in compliance with the IRS. Although numerous forms must be filed to start a business, these forms are not difficult to download and complete. It usually takes a few weeks for a response, and if you begin this process early, it should not delay the start of your practice. You can complete many other activities in the meantime.

If you will be applying to become a provider for third party payment for your services, you will want to begin the application process as soon as possible so that you can be approved as a provider within a reasonable length of time. More detailed information about how to apply to become a provider for third party payment is discussed in the chapter on financing your practice.

WORKING WITH OTHER PROFESSIONALS

It is strongly recommended that you work with a lawyer and an accountant as you establish your practice. These professionals possess skills and knowledge that you likely do not, and paying for their expertise may save you from having legal or financial problems. You will want to find someone familiar with business law to guide you through some of the forms and details of protecting yourself and your practice. One way to find a lawyer with the expertise you need is to talk to other small business owners and ask them if they have used a lawyer. Was the lawyer easy to work with? Have they been satisfied with the services provided? After you identify at least two lawyers others have found helpful, schedule an interview with each one and ask them whether they have expertise in the type of practice you are planning. An interview with a potential lawyer should not cost you anything, but you will want to inquire about fees for the work to be done for your practice. Accountants can be similarly identified and interviewed. An accountant will assist you with taxes involved in operating your private practice, a skill that most occupational therapy practitioners do not have. If you lack expertise in managing money, you may also want to hire someone to manage the practice's accounts. Solie-Johnson (2005) suggests that you may be able to save some money on legal advice by preparing your own documents and then having them reviewed by your lawyer. When you need a document, find a template for it and fill it out to the best of your ability; then consult with your lawyer about any necessary revisions.

One word of caution with regard to forming a small business relates to working with relatives. Working with a parent or a spouse can complicate relationships and lead to conflicts. It is recommended that you avoid this type of relationship. Utilizing the services of a family member would also be ill advised when hiring an accountant or a lawyer. Although these services may be free, the eventual nonmonetary cost could be very high.

WHERE WILL YOU LOCATE?

If you will not be going to your clients to provide services, they will be coming to you and you will need to find a location that meets the needs of both your service and your clients. Even if you will be going to your clients, you will still need a business office. Many community practitioners use home offices because they are convenient and offer maximum flexibility in work hours. In any case, you need a designated space that is used only for your business so that you can maintain secure and confidential client records. Having a dedicated space for a home office also can help in separation of home life from work life. You will want to budget for your home office furniture, including a desk, chair, good lighting, secured file cabinets, and bookshelves for reference materials. A computer, printer, copier, and fax are essential to any business. Having a dedicated phone line is important because you will use this to communicate with clients and to transmit billing information. As you travel from one client to another you will need to take information with you. Consider equipment that is easily portable such as a notebook computer or phone that can store information to be downloaded to your home computer. You will want to verify with an accountant which office equipment, furniture, and supplies, as well as how much office space can be considered as tax deductions. If you will be providing services in your home, you will need to check zoning ordinances in your community to be certain this is permissible.

Identify Your Needs

If you need to locate a practice space outside of your home, begin your search by specifying the amount of space you will need to accommodate your service. Be sure to include equipment, client waiting area, and office operations in your estimate. Structural building requirements may exist for special equipment, telecommunication needs, lavatory and other sanitation needs, and accessibility requirements. If most of your clients will be using wheelchairs or have ambulation difficulties, you must be sure that they can get into your practice space easily and will have access to adapted toilet facilities. Ample handicapped parking spaces close to your entrance are also required. If you will use equipment that must be ceiling or wall mounted, confirm that the building you are considering can bear the weight load of this equipment.

When you purchase a home, location is often the most important consideration. You want a home close to community resources that have value to you and your family, such as good schools, and you want your neighborhood to be safe. Similar considerations are important when you choose a location for your practice. You need your location to be convenient for your clients since many of them will be unwilling or unable to travel a distance to use your services. You can begin your location search with another visit to your public library. There you can identify trends in where people live, where they access public transportation routes, and the names of local realtors who can help you in your search. Keep in mind demographic information such as cultural characteristics, income levels, and population ages and density across different areas of your community, because all these may influence the best location for your practice. If you are located in a city with public transportation, you want to be close to a bus or other public vehicle drop-off point. Consider the time of day clients will use your service. Clients who work may want you located close to their offices; parents may prefer a location close to their home, children's school, or day care center. Cost of transportation is a factor for many people, and time is valuable. Selecting a location that minimizes client travel between home, work, and school is important.

Leasing Space

Most small businesses begin in leased space, as it offers less risk than building or purchasing an existing location (Barringer & Ireland, 2008). Once you identify the ideal space and have determined that it meets the needs of your practice and is convenient for clients, you will need to enter into a leasing agreement with the owner of the building. If you have worked with a real estate agent in locating your space, the agent will be able to help you with the lease agreement. Consider the cost of the lease, the length of the lease agreement, and any services to be provided by the owner, such as utilities, rest rooms, janitorial services, or telecommunication connections. Before you sign a lease agreement, you will want to be certain that you will have the financial resources you need to honor the agreement. This may require you to secure financing of your practice before signing a lease. You will need, however, to have a reasonable estimate of the cost of space for practice in order to prepare the budget needed for application for a business loan. This means you will need to explore your location options fairly early in your practice planning.

You may decide that your clients will be best served if you locate in an existing community services building such as a recreation center or school. Discuss your space needs with the organization in question to determine whether they are able to lease space to your practice at the times you would like to provide services to clients. Be prepared to discuss how both parties would benefit from the location of your practice in the building. Think about what you can offer the organization in return for the opportunity to lease space that may be well located and suited to your practice. An example is collaborating with a private school to lease space after school hours for services for special needs children. The children may already be at the school during the day so this would be a convenient location for parents. The space would otherwise go unused after school hours, and it accommodates your service needs. The school may benefit by providing a convenient location for services that parents want for their children, and you may be able to negotiate an opportunity to provide consultative services to the school during school hours. As you search for your location, consider how you might collaborate with others in the community, or what you might offer in exchange for getting the space you want at the most reasonable cost.

Once you decide on a location that meets your service and client needs—and have agreed with the leasing company that any needed modification can be made—you will work with a contractor to prepare the leased space for your services. Construction on leased space will follow signing of a lease. Working with contractors may be challenging and you will want to find a contractor who is reliable and has experience with similar construction projects in the community. In the same way you located a lawyer or accountant, the best way to find a contractor who will deliver quality construction that meets all local building codes and stays on schedule is to talk to others who have experienced office or home modifications. Other businesses that have undergone renovations to suit their needs, or people who have had major renovations done to their homes, may make recommendations and offer information about their experiences with their contractor. When you interview contractors, give them specific information about what you want done in your location and the types of materials you want used. Make your decision based on the estimate they prepare of time frame and costs to complete the project. If estimated costs differ significantly among contractors, ask for an explanation. Rely on the references given by others in making your decision. You will work closely with this person to select materials and design your work space; it helps to have someone you enjoy working with and whom you trust.

Buy or Build Your Own Space

You may want to build or purchase a building to use for your practice. You will have already considered that this will be a significant expense in starting your practice. In the current economic environment, a new business may have difficulty arranging financing to buy or build, and it is an additional risk to have high interest payments as you build a practice. In some cases, however, depending on the services you wish to offer, it may be best to build to accommodate special needs of your clients. You will need to adhere to local zoning laws as you search for a location. As you purchase or build a location for your practice, you will need to work with a real estate agent, a lawyer, a builder, and building inspectors. Accomplishing these tasks will take more time than if you decide to lease space already available. It is fair to say that the real estate and rental markets may play a significant role in your decision on where to locate. Working with a realtor specializing in commercial property will help you decide what is best for your practice.

Supplies and Equipment

Supplies and equipment needed to begin your practice may be either a minimal or a significant cost consideration. Make a list of all the equipment you need. Either start with a wish list and then, as you determine costs, eliminate nonessential items, or list only those things you absolutely must have to begin offering your services, and try to minimize costs as you shop for the items. If you want to start your practice with cost savings in mind, shop for used equipment on line, or see if you can negotiate a lower price with vendors in exchange for advertising their products in your practice (Barringer & Ireland, 2008). If you are going to offer driving evaluations, you need to purchase a car that can be equipped with the adaptive devices that make driving safer for people with different abilities. Buy a used car, preferably a model that is frequently driven by the types of clients you will serve, and then negotiate with vendors of adaptive devices to install their equipment on your car at a reduced price. In return, you will agree to send your clients to the provider when they need the equipment installed in their own cars. Both you and the vendor benefit from this type of arrangement. Some occupational therapy practices require fairly minimal equipment and supplies that can be purchased at discount or warehouse stores. Plan for expendable practice and office supplies such as evaluation forms, paper, printer cartridges, and other materials that once used must be replenished. Identifying, purchasing, and installing the equipment and supplies you will need to open the doors of your practice will be exciting and also produce some anxiety. You may worry about the costs you have incurred to get your practice started, or you may delight in the realization that as your office takes shape, and the equipment and supplies needed to start practice are all gathered in place, it is time to be in business for yourself.

Marks (2006) identifies reasons why small businesses do not succeed. These can include poor planning, the wrong location, poor or ineffective time management, poor customer service, or offering the wrong service. By utilizing the many resources available to assist you in planning and establishing a practice, it is possible to maximize your potential to succeed in community practice.

CHAPTER SUMMARY

This chapter is an overview of decisions you must make as you plan and establish your community practice. You need to further define your practice, justify that it meets best practice standards, and confirm that what you propose is deliverable. Deciding whether to be a solo practitioner or to partner with others is a decision with legal and tax implications; working with a legal advisor throughout the planning of your practice is a wise investment. You will clarify that your practice meets the professional regulatory requirements of your state, and that you are complying with federal and state regulations as well as local zoning requirements. You will complete your practice plans by acquiring a space that meets your own and your clients' needs, and by identifying the equipment and supplies required to start your business venture.

LEARNING ACTIVITIES

This chapter provides information that will lead to development of the following documents needed to apply for a loan or a grant:

- Mission statement
- Program plan

1. In Chapter 7, you identified a need for services to be offered in your community. Combine your interests and great ideas for a community practice with the needs you have identified, and develop them into a mission-statement for your practice. The statement should not be longer than one paragraph, following the guidelines in this chapter.
2. Your community practice should offer evaluation and interventions that have proven to be effective. Prepare a tentative list of interventions you would like to offer clients and search for evidence of the effectiveness of each.

   Justify the inclusion of each intervention you will offer in your practice by citing research that supports its efficacy.

   Develop a short narrative describing your practice. Describe the clients you will serve, their needs, and the interventions that have proven effective in addressing those needs. Cite evidence to support your decision to offer those interventions.
3. Get a copy of your state practice regulations and verify that each intervention planned for your practice is allowable professional practice in your state.
4. Create a plan describing how you will operate your program, including location, hours of operation, and staff requirements. Justify each of these decisions based on community culture, client needs, and opportunities for your practice to be successful in an environment where competition may exist.
5. Choose a name for your practice following guidelines suggested in this chapter. Determine whether this name would be allowed if you chose to incorporate your practice in your state.
6. Location of your practice needs to be convenient for clients. In identifying a location, you need to seek out space that will be compatible with the types of intervention you plan to offer and clients you plan to serve. List all factors that must go into selecting a location for your

specific program. Estimate the amount of space needed to provide each type of intervention, office space needed to administer the practice, and sufficient space for client reception and waiting area. Is the space accessible to your clients? Can you find a location that meets your specifications? What is the amount you would need to budget for rental of this location?

7. List any modifications that would need to be made to your location to accommodate your practice. List all equipment needed to provide the evaluations and interventions you plan to offer clients. List equipment you will need to furnish your office, as well as reception and waiting area. List expendable supplies such as testing materials, office supplies, and other consumable products such as cleaning materials. This list will be used to develop a program budget in the next chapter.

REFERENCES

Addy., L. (2006). *Occupational therapy evidence in practice for physical rehabilitation.* Malden, MA: Blackwell Publishing.

American Occupational Therapy Association (2008). Occupational therapy practice framework: Domain and Process (2nd ed.). *The American Journal of Occupational Therapy, 62* (6) 625–683.

Bailey, D.M., Bornstein, J. & Ryan, S. (2007). A case report of evidence-based practice: From academia to clinic. *The American Journal of Occupational Therapy, 61* (1) 85–91.

Barringer, B.R. & Ireland, R.D. (2008). *What's stopping you? Shatter the 9 most common myths keeping you from starting your own business.* Upper Saddle River, NJ: Pearson Education, Inc.

Bennett, S., Hoffman, T., McCluskey, A., McKenna, K., Strong, J., & Tooth, L. (2003). Introducing OTseeker (Occupational therapy systematic evaluation): A new evidence database for occupational therapists. *The American Journal of Occupational Therapy, 57* (6) 635–638.

Corcoran, M. (2006). From the desk of the editor: A busy practitioner's approach to evidence-based practice. *The American Journal of Occupational Therapy, 60* (2) 127–128.

Kotler, P., Hayes, T. & Bloom, P.N. (2002). Marketing Professional Services (2nd ed.). NJ: Prentice Hall

Law, M.C. & MacDermid, J. (2008). *Evidence-based rehabilitation: A guide to practice.* Thorofare, NJ: Slack, Inc.

Long, C. & Cronin-Davis, J. (2006). *Occupational therapy evidence in practice for mental health.* Malden, MA: Blackwell Publishing.

Mancuso, A. (2007). *How to form a non-profit corporation* (8th ed.). Berkeley, CA: Nolo.

Marks, G. (2006). *Small business book of lists.* Avon MA: Adams Media.

McKenna, K., Bennett, S., Dierselhuis, Z., Hoffman, L, Tooth, L. & McCluskey, A. (2005). Australian occupational therapists' use of an online evidence-based practice database (OTseeker). *Health Information & Libraries Journal, 22* (3) 205–214.

Pakroo, P.H. (2008). *The small business start-up kit: A step by step legal guide* (5th ed.). Berkeley, CA: Nolo.

Peters, T.C. (2005). *Re-imagine! Business excellence in a disruptive age.* London: Dorling Kindersley, Ltd.

Polatajko, H.J. & Craik, J. (2006). In search of evidence: Strategies for an evidence-based practice process. *Occupational Therapy Journal of Research, 26* (1) 2–3.

Solie-Johnson, K. (2005) *How to set up your own small business.* Minneapolis, MN: American Institute of Small Business.

Stephenson, J. & Mintzer, R. (2008). *Ultimate homebased business handbook* (2nd ed.) Madison, WI: CWL Publishing.

RESOURCES

American Occupational Therapy Association, Evidence-Based Practice Resource Directory.
> http://www.aota.org. Retrieved December 11, 2008.

Cumulative index to nursing and allied health literature (CINAHL).
> http://www.CINAHL.com. Retrieved December 11, 2008.

Internal Revenue Service (IRS).
> http://www.irs.gov. Retrieved December 11, 2008.

OTseeker. International database of occupational therapy resources.
> http://www.otseeker.com.

Federal government database of registered business names.
> http://www.business.gov/register/business-name/naming.htm. Retrieved December 11, 2008.

InterNIC-Public information regarding internet domain name registration services.
> http://www.internic.com. Retrieved December 11, 2008.

Service Corps of Retired Executives (SCORE).
> http://www.score.org. Retrieved December 11, 2008.

Small Business Development Center.
> http://www.sba.gov/sbdc. Retrieved December 9, 2008.

U.S. Chamber of Commerce.
> http://uschamber.com. Retrieved December 10, 2008.

Chapter 9

Financing Your Practice

LEARNING OBJECTIVES

- Prepare budget and other materials needed to obtain funding for your practice.
- Select potential sources of financing to start and maintain your practice.
- Develop economic strategies to succeed in community practice.

INTRODUCTION

This chapter will explain how to develop a budget you will use for multiple purposes, including planning your business, approaching lenders, and monitoring your practice. Identifying potential loan sources and preparing to work with lenders will be necessary if you will require external funding to get your practice started. Grants, as a potential source of start-up funding, require special consideration and careful preparation. Maintaining financial support for your practice includes identifying sources of revenue production.

FINANCIAL PLANNING

In planning a new business venture, one major concern is financial resources. You likely will be spending more money than you are receiving in income during the first months of a new practice. When compared to assurances of a steady paycheck from an employer, thinking about financial insecurity can produce anxiety. Developing realistic financial plans, however, should provide reassurance that you will recover your initial costs and be financially successful as your business develops over time. There are different ways of financing a new practice, and costs will vary depending on the type of practice planned and the potential sources of payment for your services.

Some community programs provided in recent years were initially developed at minimal or no cost to the developers by utilizing volunteers and existing resources. Often these programs were provided as community service by students or others who were not depending on the program for their personal income. Volunteer programs often end after a specific period of time because students or other volunteers do not remain available to provide services. If these programs have been beneficial to clients, an agency may want to continue providing services. Funding will be needed to hire people to replace some or all of the volunteers and to cover other costs of the program. For example, many aging-in-place programs began as opportunities to bring occupational therapy students and supervising faculty members together with aging adults to address a community need for elders to be safely independent in their homes. These programs usually began with a faculty member who identified an agency providing services to aging adults living independently, and made arrangements for supervised students to provide home assessments and recommendations to improve safe independent living. Services, which are provided with no monetary exchanges by any participants, yield nonmonetary benefits to all participants. Student programs are limited, however, by availability of students and their supervisor's availability to arrange and supervise student services. If an aging-in-place program is successful and the collaborating senior services organization wants to continue offering services, they may hire an occupational therapy practitioner to provide them.

As you initiate your new community practice, part of your business plan will involve projecting the initial expenses you will incur to start offering your services, projecting the costs to stay in business for a year, and anticipating the revenue generated by your first year of practice. Understanding financial management of your resources is necessary to apply for a loan, to meet tax requirements, and to satisfy yourself and your clients that you are providing value with your services. Financial plans will be built on a process that begins with the foundation of ideas you developed from talking to community members and acquiring evidence of best practice. Ideas and plans then become monetary objectives for your practice. In developing financial plans, you will have considered where you will locate your practice, whether you will be providing all services yourself or hiring others, what equipment and supplies you will need to get started, and how your program will continue to operate over time. You could approach financial planning by envisioning your ideal practice, or by limiting yourself to what you can afford to offer when you begin practice. If you choose the latter, you can plan to expand as your business succeeds and your financial situation improves. Barringer and Ireland (2008) suggest that frugality in starting a business yields success because owners focus on becoming self-reliant and operating within their means as they strive to meet clients' needs. Another reason to be frugal is that when the national economy is contracting, it may be more difficult to borrow money. Good ideas that provide needed services may still find funding, however, if the business owners can prove they have used restraint in developing realistic budgets.

Financial planning can be done alone or with others, such as partners in practice or an accountant. If you will be working with others in your practice, you may want to involve them in the financial planning process. Having more than one person involved provides opportunity for discussion of what is needed for practice as well as ways to minimize costs. Whether you plan alone or with others, you must be realistic in your plans so that whatever expense you propose is essential and you are certain that money you borrow will be spent as allocated.

You will need to prepare different types of financial plans, including projected costs to start your practice, an income statement that gives cost and revenue projections for one year, a cash flow statement that projects how much cash you are likely to have each month to pay expenses, and a balance sheet that lists your total assets and liabilities as a measure of the value of your practice. When you start your practice, you will need to project these budgets for the first year of operations, but in following years, you will use actual financial data from the previous year (Pakroo, 2008). Lenders will want to see costs of everything, especially in challenging economic times when investors want to be fairly certain that they will receive a return on their investment.

Start-Up Costs

Begin financial planning by projecting costs needed to start your business. The U.S. Chamber of Commerce provides a library of resources to assist in starting a small business, including a work sheet to estimate the cost of start-up. Examples of expenses you may incur in starting your business include the purchase or lease of space and equipment, initial inventory costs of therapy and office supplies, furnishings, assets and personal liability insurance, utilities, advertising, licenses and fees, and professional costs for consulting with an attorney or an accountant. For each service you plan to offer, identify any supplies or equipment needed and identify the actual cost to purchase or lease these materials.

Income Statement: Fixed and Variable Costs

Costs associated with a budget cycle or a year of practice will need to be projected for your first year of operations. There are two types of costs to consider in your projections. Fixed costs include the bills that you have to pay no matter how many clients you see; variable costs are costs that fluctuate with the volume of your business. Fixed costs include rent, utilities, payment for equipment purchased or rented, liability and property insurance, and any other services that are required for you to stay in practice no matter how many clients you have. You will have to pay these costs whether you provide services to two or twenty clients each day. Variable costs, on the other hand, include supplies or anything else that fluctuates with the number of clients served. Salaries and benefits may be either fixed or variable costs depending on whether they fluctuate with the quantity of services provided. If you plan to be in a solo practice and provide services only to the number of clients you can manage on your own, your salary and benefits are fixed. If, however, you are hoping your practice will grow and you will need to hire additional service providers to meet needs of increasing numbers of clients, these costs would be variable. You will also need to project revenue from your practice. Revenue is the payment you expect to receive from your clients for the services you provide. If your annual income exceeds your costs you will be profitable; if costs exceed income you will be operating at a loss.

Cash Flow Projections

Monthly cash flow projections will show how much cash you are likely to have compared to monthly debt. Utilizing the categories identified for your income statement, you will project costs and revenues for each month. When you first open your practice, your costs most likely will exceed your revenue and you will have a negative cash flow. As time passes, however, you will expect revenue to exceed costs to a break-even point in order to stay in business. A cash flow statement is required when seeking a business loan because lenders are looking for investments that eventually will produce profit, or loans that can be repaid with interest.

Direct and Indirect Expenses

In developing a budget that covers your first year of operations, categorizing your expenses as direct or indirect can provide you with tax advantages (Pakroo, 2008). Indirect expenses are those costs associated with business operations that are shared with another function, such as a home office or car payments on a car used for personal as well as business purposes. You will need to assign a percentage of business use and personal use for each item you classify as an indirect expense. If you are working with an accountant to set up your practice, this person can help you establish your indirect expenses and will also be sure your business is in compliance with federal and state tax regulations.

Direct expenses can be fully deducted from your taxes and include personnel needed to implement your practice. In a budget, personnel costs are reported as FTEs (full time equivalent) payments. A full-time, or 40-hour-a-week, employee is 1FTE. Someone working 10 hours a week is .25 FTE. If you are planning for full-time employment, you will need to include the expense of benefits such as health insurance, social security, unemployment and disability insurance, vacation, and holidays. Salary expenses for personnel vary with location because salaries are based partly on supply and demand. Professional salaries are often available from the results of surveys done by professional organizations. The American Occupational Therapy Association (AOTA) reports salary survey results through its Web site. Benefits are usually calculated at 30% of salary costs, but you will want to try to calculate these benefits as close to actual costs as possible. Even if you are to be the only employee, you need to project the cost of your salary. If you will be using part-time employees, you may want to project an hourly rate in your budget (a variable or fixed cost) that may not include benefits. If taxes are not withheld for hourly workers, these persons are responsible for paying those taxes to federal and state governments. Any contract with employees will specify responsibility for tax payments. Verify with an accountant the tax requirements and consequences involved with hiring employees.

Capital equipment includes items that cost enough to depreciate over time. There are different thresholds for depreciating equipment based on original cost and life span. You will want to review IRS regulations by reading their publications on the topic, which can be downloaded from their Web site. You also may wish to discuss capital equipment costs and depreciation with your accountant. Some occupational therapy equipment may qualify for this tax deduction based on cost and life span; verify with your accountant whether this applies to your practice. If what you need to operate your program does not qualify for the equipment category, you probably will need to identify it as a supply. Supplies include anything under the cost threshold for equipment that you need to implement your activities in your practice. If you need to modify existing structures to offer your program, you will need to budget for construction costs, which may include mounting ceiling hooks for swings, constructing ramps for therapy, and modifying a building to be accessible.

Communication costs include telecommunications services and equipment dedicated to your practice. If you need them for your program and they are not otherwise available, their cost is tax deductible. If you are working from a home office, communication costs will be an indirect expense unless you add a dedicated line solely for business purposes. Other items you might include in your direct budget are rent for the space to operate your program and marketing activities.

When your budget is prepared and you are comfortable that all of your expenses are justified, you are ready to search for external funding to get your practice started.

In order to apply for a loan you will need to provide a cash flow statement, an income statement, a balance sheet, and a personal financial statement that states your net worth based on personal assets and liabilities. The Small Business Administration (SBA) Web site provides instruction about how to prepare financial statements required in a loan package.

ESTABLISHING A PRICE FOR YOUR SERVICES

Setting fees for your program is one of the more challenging tasks of establishing a new service, but will be necessary in order to prepare financial statements. The three methods most often used in establishing fees for professional services that are to be paid for privately are:

- Cost-oriented method
- Time and expense method
- Competition-oriented method

If you expect to be paid for your services by third-party payers, your fee likely is set by payer policy. You should explore the rate of reimbursement in order to determine if your practice is feasible at this rate. The option you choose for payment—private or third-party—may limit the expenses you can incur in setting up your practice and will determine the revenue you can expect for your services.

Cost-Oriented Method

The cost-oriented method requires fees to be based on the actual costs to deliver the service. To these you would then add an additional cost, which is your profit. The cost for services would include all of the costs projected in your income statement: personnel costs plus benefits, rent or location costs and overhead, supplies and equipment, and preparation and follow-up services. The total of these costs would be divided by the number of hours of service you project would be available. This would result in a per-hour cost that you would then charge for individual services.

If you will be offering services that group clients together for the best outcome, you would divide your hourly cost by the number of clients seen in each group to arrive at a cost for group therapy. If costs are to be reimbursed in total or in part by third-party payers, different rates would need to be established for individual and group treatments, and in some cases group treatment would not be allowed. If some of your services require more time, supplies, or equipment than other services, you may have different prices for each service you offer. If you are in an area where there is no reasonable competition, and you are not going to be constrained by prices set by third-party payers, you will use the cost-oriented method to establish your fees. You need to keep in mind, however, that clients will seek your services based on their ability to pay and their perception of the value of your services. This is where knowing your market is essential. What people want or need and their economic ability to pay for it will determine the success or failure of your practice.

Time and Expense Method

Similar to the cost-oriented method of setting fees is the time and expense method. This sets an hourly rate according to what is reasonable and customary in your area, and adds additional expenses, such as supplies, equipment, or travel costs, to the established amount. If you will be working alone and taking services to clients, this may be the preferred method of establishing your fees for service. Needless to say, there can be a wide range of fees locally. An example would be a fee paid for services provided to children. These payments may range from a flat $25 an hour fee for a home visit for a child on Medicaid to a charge of $250 for an hour of therapy delivered in a hospital outpatient setting in which the actual hourly amount paid to the therapist is $30 to $40. The hospital based charge reflects overhead expense associated with use of the hospital facility.

Competition-Oriented Method

Another method you might use to set fees for your service is the competition-oriented method. In this method you would attempt to find practices similar to your own and find out what they are charging for their services. It would be desirable to find several competitors with similar services who have higher and lower prices and then try to position your own fees somewhere in the middle. You can hope to attract some clients away from competitors with lower prices, yet still have fees that allow self-sustaining operation of your practice. If you price your services much above the cost of similar services, potential clients may go to the lower priced option and you will need to adjust prices downward to attract clients. Conversely, if you set your prices much lower than the competition, clients may perceive that your lower prices reflect less value and choose to follow their perceptions that the higher priced competition is preferable to your services.

Setting prices is based on the economic principle of supply and demand. When supply is greater than demand, services are discounted to attract more clients; when demand for services is greater than what can be supplied, prices rise as clients will pay a premium to have what they want or need. Price setting is an important part of your marketing strategy and one where client perception is important. Desire for a service, plus perception of quality and convenience, determine what clients are willing to pay for services.

FINDING MONEY TO START YOUR PRACTICE

Some individuals have personal resources to start a practice, but Solie-Johnson (2005) suggests financing your business with other people's money in order to share the risk. This may make sense for some, but for others borrowing money leads to additional worries about repayment of loans, shared management, or shared decision making. You may need to consider external financing for at least part of your practice start-up costs if you do not have the personal resources to finance your own practice. You do not want to be underfunded since this often leads to business failure if you cannot sustain your payments during the early and often leaner days of a new business (Solie-Johnson, 2005).

Loans

You may seek funds either as a personal loan or from a lending institution. If you are planning a personal loan you will probably be borrowing from relatives or friends. Alternatively you would request your funding from commercial banks, small business investment companies, or community development organizations. Although going to relatives or friends may seem the easier route to financing, Green (2003) recommends that family involvement in your business is not ideal as this can lead to conflicts of interest or control issues. Depending on how much money you will need to borrow and current economic pressures, your best bet for financing is to work with the SBA to identify and plan for a loan. The SBA does not grant loans, but will assist you in securing a loan from a bank or other lender.

Keep in mind when searching for financing that you cannot get 100 percent financing and there are no government sources of free money to start a small business. Once you decide to pursue a loan from a bank or other lending institution, you will have costs associated with the loan, the same as if you borrowed money to purchase a home. You will pay loan fees in order for money to be delivered to you, followed by closing costs, attorney fees, appraisal costs to confirm the value of your loan, and possibly recording costs if you have purchased a building. Interest rates are calculated according to the risk associated with your loan; therefore, the greater the risk, the more expensive the cost of the loan.

Whether or not you can obtain a loan, and what it will cost you, is determined by your own credit history. When you apply for a loan you will need to provide your credit history to determine the interest rate you will pay and whether you are a good investment for the lending organization. Green (2003) suggests that although big banks are able to obtain cheaper funds than smaller banks, and could offer a lower borrowing rate, it is more difficult to borrow from big banks. Newer, local, and smaller banks may be more responsive to your financial needs but loans there will cost a bit more than at larger banks.

Establishing Credit

Financing your practice also allows you to establish credit for your business, which may have future benefits. In order to keep your credit rating good, you will need to pay your bills on time. Use of a credit card has become widely accepted as a method of payment for services. The same financial institution that issues the loan for your practice may also be able to arrange for clients to pay for their services by credit card. Once you have secured your loan, you will continue to have a working relationship with your lending institution. It will expect periodic financial reports related to your original budget proposal. Having a good relationship with a financial institution can have many benefits as you develop your practice.

The SBA provides information about how to finance your practice and resources for loans at their Web site. Online instructions available there include templates for creating documents you will need to apply for a loan, preparation for meeting with a potential lender, and additional suggestions for finding a loan to meet your needs.

CONTINUING TO STAY IN BUSINESS

You will need to generate a continuous stream of income for your practice in order to meet your financial obligations and to stay in business. There are multiple sources of revenue for practice including private payment by your clients, third-party payment, contracts with other agencies in your community, and grants. There are challenges to each of these types of payment. You will want to explore the options carefully to decide if you want to rely on one source, or on multiple sources of payment for your services.

Locating your community practice in an area of economic stability and offering services that are highly desired by a segment of that community able to pay privately has many advantages. Your clients will pay what they feel is a fair price for your services, so establishing this amount will be very important to your success. Fees that are consistent with what others are charging for similar services is a good start. You can also, however, survey potential clients to determine a reasonable threshold for paying for customized services specific to their needs. You may decide to accept cash payment only, but with a community practice you are likely to have clients who prefer to pay using a credit card. You may want to make arrangements for credit card payments before opening your practice.

Keep in mind that if you choose to accept only private payment, this may limit the clients you can accept. You may want to consider developing a sliding scale for those clients less financially able to pay your fees, or decide to accept a mix of private and third-party payments. If services are directed toward children, those living in less affluent socioeconomic areas may be limited to services reimbursed through a government supported system, whereas children living in areas of greater affluence may have parents who will pay whatever they think your services are worth to their children. If you are planning services for aging adults, Peters (2005) states that these clients often have financial resources to purchase whatever they want or need, so private payment may be their preferred payment method.

Collaborating with other organizations to offer services that are needed by clients in your community provides another option for financial stability of your practice. Such an arrangement would immediately minimize your risk of starting a community practice because you could develop a contract with the collaborating agency that specified and assured a set payment for the services that you deliver. Sometimes, having a contract with an organization is a good method of ensuring some job security as you continue developing a private practice dependent on other forms of payment. If your goal is future independent practice, however, you need to be cautious about signing noncompetitive agreements with the organization; doing so would make it difficult for you to remain in the community in direct competition with a former employer.

Payment by Third Parties

Third-party payments are desirable when the services you plan to provide are typically covered by health insurance. Before proceeding to become a third-party payer service provider, you will need to verify that what you plan to offer is covered by the payer and that you qualify as a service provider of that service in your state. Occupational therapy scope of practice as specified in the occupational therapy practice framework and state practice regulations will identify what services you can perform for third-party reimbursement (AOTA, 2008; Slater & Willmarth, 2005). If you are planning to practice with aging adults, your potential clients may qualify for payment through Medicare. This will require you to be in compliance with Medicare regulations. If you will be offering services to low income clients, they may qualify for Medicaid payments. Each state administers its own Medicaid program; you will need to contact your state to determine whether your services would qualify for payment and how to bill for your services.

Becoming a State or National Provider of Health Care Services

To receive Medicare or Medicaid reimbursement for your services, you must enroll as a service provider through a national registry for covered healthcare providers. To do this, you must have a National Provider Identifier (NPI). The NPI was developed to improve efficiency and effectiveness in electronic transmission of health information. You apply for your NPI online at the National Plan and Provider Enumeration System Web site. This Web site provides additional information about billing for your services. After you receive your NPI you can complete an online application at the same Web site to enroll as a Medicare service provider.

Grant Funding

Types of Grants

A grant is a gift, usually of money, for a specific purpose. Organizations or government agencies have money to invest in programs or research consistent with their values and priorities. Granting organizations set the parameters of the projects they are willing to fund as well as the amount they will invest in each project they determine meets their criteria for funding. Organizations award different types of grants, therefore you will want to match your need to the type of grant offered. Some project grants fund a program cycle, other grants provide money only to start up a program, and fewer grants will provide operating funds for an established program. Challenge grants require you to match funds with other sources to fully fund your program. If you plan to pursue grant funding for all or part of the cost for your program, you will need to correlate your needs with the type of funding an organization will provide.

Nonprofit Organization or a Collaborator

Grants have often been a source of startup money for community practices associated with universities because most grant recipients must qualify as a nonprofit 501-(c)-(3) organization according to specifications set by the Internal Revenue Service (IRS). A nonprofit organization exists to serve a mission of public interest rather than produce a profit for its directors. A nonprofit 501-(c)-3 organization must have a mission, vision, statement of bylaws, and a board of directors. To acquire this tax status, an organization must submit a request to the IRS and meet stringent requirements for use of resources.

If status as a nonprofit organization is something that fits with the community practice you are interested in starting, an excellent resource to follow is *How to Form a Nonprofit Corporation, 8th edition* (Mancuso, 2007). On the other hand, if your ideas for practice seem to support community services offered by a nonprofit organization already in your community, you might want to contact the director of that organization and see if you can collaborate by writing a grant to cover the cost of adding your services to the organization's activities. Potential collaborators might include a school or preschool, sports program, senior center, homeless shelter, community mental health program, or religious organization. Determine that your missions, clients served, and visions are compatible before approaching a potential collaborator with your ideas.

When you meet, you will need to articulate your planned program and describe how your services support and enhance the work of the nonprofit organization. Discuss compatibility of missions and program activities; then provide a tentative budget and some suggestions for potential grants to fund the program. Numerous books are available that can help identify potential grants and explain the best way to go about getting your project funded. Two of these books are: *Getting Grants: The Complete Manual of Proposal Development and Administration* (Carter-Black, 2006) and *The Only Grantwriting Book You'll Ever Need, 2nd edition* (Karsh & Fox, 2006).

When starting a practice with a grant, your collaborator will want to have assurance that your program will continue when grant funds are no longer available. Few grants continue over an extended period of time, yet in order to receive a grant your program must be considered important to a community. Consequently, you will need to show how you will continue to fund your program beyond a grant funded period. Possibilities for future funding include fees paid privately or by third-party payment. If you are planning to provide services to low income clients, you may want to consider applying for a nonprofit status for your practice, independent of your original collaborator. Obtaining this status will enable you to raise funds to offset the costs of providing services to clients who may be unable to pay.

Identifying Potential Grants

Private and corporate foundations, along with local agencies, are the likeliest sources of grants for community programs that offer services to meet specific needs of residents. The most important thing to remember when searching for grant money to fund your program is that grants are not about you, not about money, and not about gifts; grants are given to further the mission and vision of the grant making organization. Finding a grant for your program requires matching your needs to the grant makers' interests. Private foundations will state their current interests and funding priorities on their Web sites. They may identify projects recently funded, which may help you determine whether your program is consistent with their interests. The Foundation Center Web site and other Web sites offer access to databases of organizations offering grants. Through these databases you can search for grants that seem to match your program needs.

One way to find local grants is to do a "Google" search for community foundations or grants by city or state. Corporations and businesses frequently fund projects that improve quality of life for their workers and other residents of their community. You can locate these potential funding sources through the corporate Web site or through a listing of foundations specific to your location.

Foundations and other grant making organizations usually provide guidelines for inquiry about their grants. Most often this requires a short application or a letter of inquiry that describes your proposal and your qualifications. Some foundations are responsive to phone calls or e-mail messages, whereas others will be unresponsive to these personal contacts. Generally speaking, local organizations are more likely to welcome personal contact. Larger foundations with more money to fund projects, and consequently more applications for grants, limit contact with applicants to the forms or letters specified in their guidelines. Some foundations review letters of inquiry or brief applications first in order to winnow applicants from many to only a few who will submit full-length grant proposals.

Grant Application

Once you have matched your program with the mission and vision of a potential funding source, you will need to prepare a grant application. This will be your opportunity to show your worth to a potential grant provider through a linear plan demonstrating how you will help them fulfill their mission. Your plan needs to be easy to read and understand, and must address the needs and priorities of the granting organization. It should also prove to them that you have sufficient management skills to successfully implement the project.

Upon receiving a grant application, read it carefully and organize the materials you need to complete and submit the application. You will need to provide the following information: your program/organization name, letter of tax exemption, years your organization has been in existence, names of applicants and contact information, amount of money you are requesting, type of request (e.g., startup or technical assistance), the period the grant will cover, project title, and total project and organization budgets. You will also provide your mission statement and summarize the program or project you would like funded. Some foundations may review this brief overview as a separate document and as a precursor to a complete grant application. For others it may accompany a completed application. Grant providers review the non-narrative details of your application to determine whether your project meets their requirements and whether they are interested in potentially funding it.

A full grant application will include pre-narrative forms, an abstract or executive summary of your program, information about your organization, and a statement describing the need for your program, its design, and plans for operation and evaluation. Financial information required in a grant application includes an overall program budget, your specific monetary request, and a description of how this money will be used. Chapter 8 provides information you need to prepare a statement of need for your program and its purpose, design, and justification. This chapter describes how to develop a budget, and Chapter 11 provides specific information about developing program evaluation. When writing the history of your organization, identify its major accomplishments related to the program for which you are seeking a grant. Show how the population you serve with your program mirrors the populations that the funding organization has supported in current or recent funding cycles. Often foundations are looking for collaboration within a community of other nonprofit and for-profit groups.

Packaging the Grant for Submission

Your application for a grant may be accompanied by a cover letter to a foundation director. The letter should reflect your understanding of the foundation's mission and interests correlated with your program's objectives. The letter should not be an executive summary of your program, but rather an opportunity to form a personal connection with the foundation. Before you send your application, carefully review the grant requirements and what you have provided in your proposal. It is always a good idea to have another person review your materials to look for inconsistencies or omissions. The smallest detail can often derail a proposal from being funded. Make sure that all required documents are attached and in the order required by the foundation. Present the completed document as instructed. Note whether staples or bindings are allowed. Provide the number of copies requested and keep one copy for your records. Be sure your proposal is postmarked before the deadline and use a postage method that provides evidence of date of mailing and date of arrival.

Outcomes of Grant Applications

Once the grant has been mailed, the average time before notification of results is six months for corporate grants and one year for foundations. During this time, you may receive a request for additional information, or a site visit by a foundation officer. Either event may mean you are on a short list of proposals for funding. You will want to provide whatever additional information is needed to demonstrate your ability to successfully achieve your program objectives and be responsive to the foundation. Most foundations are unresponsive to phone calls or other efforts by your organization to gain information about what is happening with your grant proposal.

If your program is funded, you will likely receive notification by phone, followed by a letter stating the amount of the grant and requesting information from you to facilitate the transfer of funds to your organization's account. This letter will further state the requirements for accountability of the money granted your organization.

The chance of not being funded is significant given that the average success rate is one in ten applications. A couple of factors can increase the odds of your success. One, you have been successful in receiving previous grant awards. Two, you have employed a professional grant writer to prepare your grant application. If the date of announcements of grant awards has passed and you have not received notification, you may be able to check the foundation Web site for a list of awards or you may phone the foundation to ask if decisions have been made. Most awardees are phoned and if a grant is not awarded, you receive a letter.

Most foundations and other grant providers fund only about 10% to 20% of all applications they receive. Even experienced grant writers see only about one-quarter of their submitted projects funded. Given this reality of grant funding success, you must not feel defeated, but accept this as a learning opportunity. Review the copy of your proposal and compare it once more with the request for proposals, and look critically at what they wanted and what you submitted. Was your proposal clear and compelling? Did you follow guidelines and answer every question? Did you leave anything out? Did your budget make sense and was it in line with usual grant amounts given by the foundation? Were there computational errors or was narrative poorly written? Some grant providers will offer reviewer comments, but others merely will refer you to the review process. If you do not receive written feedback on your proposal, phone the foundation and ask if you may reapply in another grant cycle and how you might improve your proposal. Listen carefully, make notes, don't interrupt, and never be defensive when receiving feedback. Always use whatever feedback you receive, whether you plan to resubmit your proposal or apply for different grant.

CHAPTER SUMMARY

It is desirable to work collaboratively with others in establishing a budget and identifying future funding sources for your program. Even if you have decided to establish a solo practice, you may want to have assistance in planning for the implementation and management of your business. Talking to others who have experience in starting their own practice or a small business will help you identify tips for success and pitfalls to avoid. While a lawyer is very helpful in preparing your business structure, an accountant can be beneficial in planning the financial structure of your business. Having an accountant with expertise gained from working with other small businesses could save you considerable frustration in the future. He will also help you examine the tax implications of various business structures, as well as let you know what to expect regarding annual and quarterly tax obligations.

You will need to immerse yourself in developing, justifying, understanding, and explaining a budget for your practice. Identifying and approaching individuals or institutions to seek funding for practice requires you to explain your budget confidently to others and convince them of your ability to succeed as a business. Deciding on the best approach to sustaining your practice through payments for your services will be important not only to you but to your investors. One of the reasons for starting your own community practice is to be self-supporting and make money while meeting community needs. Taking time to understand the financial aspects of your practice is time well spent.

Grants may be a source of financing to start a program but you will need to comply with requirements of foundations or other organizations that issue grants. Establishing a nonprofit organization or collaborating with a community organization that is already a nonprofit organization, while tirelessly adhering to grant application guidelines, may lead to successful funding.

LEARNING ACTIVITIES

These activities are designed to guide your production of financial documents necessary for financing you practice through a loan or a grant:

- Budget of costs necessary to start your practice
- Income statement
- Cash flow statement

1. Estimating the costs to start your practice begins by itemizing everything you need to open your doors to your first clients. In Chapter 8 you listed location, equipment, furniture, and supplies needed. Add to this list costs for insurance, utilities, advertising, license fees, consultation fees, salary, and benefits costs. Assign an actual cost for each item.

   Classify each cost as fixed or variable. Fixed costs are those costs you pay whether you have any clients or not; for example, a rental agreement for one year is a fixed monthly cost each month of the contract. Variable costs fluctuate with the number of clients you serve. To start your practice, budget for only the amount of these materials you need for clients expected when you start practice.

   Further classify each item as a direct or indirect cost. Indirect costs are associated with items that you use part-time for your business, such as your car or your home office. Direct expenses are those costs that are purely business expenses and are tax deductible. Deductible expenses on indirect costs are a percentage of the total cost that is used exclusively for business purposes.

   To assist you in identifying all potential costs, you may want to use the initial cash requirements worksheet developed by the Small Business Administration.

2. Establish a fee for your services. Choose the method you plan to use to set prices, such as a price comparable to your competitors or an amount that can be expected from third-party payers. Explain why

you chose the method and what your actual pricing is. Will you charge everyone the same amount? Or will amount vary by type of service provided? Explain your decision.

3. Prepare an income statement, which is the amount you expect to receive from client payments for services each month. Take into consideration how your clients will pay for services (i.e., private pay versus third-party reimbursement) and how this may affect your income. How will payment methods affect the amount of money you need to start your practice?

4. A cash flow statement reports your monthly costs and revenue for one year. Using the figures developed for your startup costs and the income you expect to receive from clients, project an income for 12 months. This statement of projected costs and revenue will be required in loan applications because the lending agency will want to see that you can recover your initial and ongoing costs with revenue. The first months, revenue will be lower than costs, but as your clients increase, you should reach a break-even point.

    You may want to graph your costs and revenues for each month during the first year to illustrate your break-even point.

5. Consider whether or not you would like to receive grant funding to start your practice. Will it be feasible for you to develop your practice as a nonprofit 501(c)(3) organization?

    If you think that starting a nonprofit organization would not be the best way to start your practice, identify a nonprofit organization in your community that would collaborate with you in seeking grant funding for your program.

    Using the organization's mission statement and other supporting information regarding its vision, clients, and services, prepare a summary of why your program is compatible and how you might enhance the organization's services to the community.

6. Identify a funding source for your program. How did you find this grant provider? How does your program support the mission and priorities of the grant provider? Review the procedures for applying for a grant and prepare a narrative describing your program and what links it with the priorities of the grant provider.

REFERENCES

American Occupational Therapy Association (AOTA). (2008). Occupational therapy practice framework: Domain and process (2nd ed.) *The American Journal of Occupational Therapy, 62* (6) 625–683.

Barringer, B.R. & Ireland, R.D. (2008). *What's stopping you? Shatter the 9 most common myths keeping you from starting your own business.* Upper Saddle River, NJ: Pearson Education Inc.

Carter-Black, A. (2006). *Getting grants: The complete manual of proposal development and administration.* Bellingham, WA: Self-Counsel Press.

Pakroo, P.H. (2008). *The small business start-up kit.* Berkeley, CA: Nolo.

Peters, T.C. (2005). *Re-imagine! Business excellence in a disruptive age.* London: Doring Kindersley, Ltd.

Green, C.H. (2003). *Financing the small business.* Aron, MA: Adams Media Corp.

Karsh, E. & Fox, A.S. (2006). *The only grant-writing book you'll ever need* (2nd ed.) NY: Carroll & Graf Publishers.

Mancuso, A. (2007). *How to form a non-profit corporation* (8th ed.) Berkeley, CA: Nolo.

Slater, D.Y. & Willmarth, C. (2005). Understanding and asserting the occupational therapy scope of practice. *OT Practice, 10* (19) CE 1–8.

Solie-Johnson, K. (2005). *How to set up your own small business.* Minneapolis, MN: American Institute of Small Business.

ELECTRONIC RESOURCES

Financial planning

American Occupational Therapy Association (AOTA) salary survey
http://www.aota.org

Small Business Development Center for free online training to start a small business
http://www.sba.gov/sbdc

Small Business Administration advice on financing a practice and locating resources for loans
http://www.sba.gov/financing. Retrieved December 14, 2008.

Small Business Administration financial planning advice
http://www.app/.sba.gov/training/sbafp

Small Business Administration initial cash requirements work sheet
http://www.uschamber.com/tools/cashne_m.asp

How to prepare a loan package
http://www.sba.gov/training/sbalp. Retrieved December 14, 2008.

United States Chamber of Commerce small business resources:
http://uschamber.com/sb. Retrieved December 14, 2008.

Service Corps of Retired Executives
http://score.org

Loan sources
http://sbdcnet.org/SBIC/finance.php

Enrolling as a service provider

To obtain an NPI number through National Plan & Provider Enumeration System:

http://NPPES.cms.hhs.gov

To enroll as a Medicare provider

http://www.cms.hhs.gov/cmsforms/downloads/cms855a.pdf. Retrieved December 12, 2008.

Taxes

http://www.irs.gov. Retrieved December 12, 2008.

Grants Available

Foundation Center. Database of organizations offering grants

http://www.fdcenter.org. Retrieved December 12, 2008.

Comprehensive list of grants available

http://www.fundsnetservices.com. Retrieved December 12, 2008.

Chapter 10

Marketing Your Program

- Apply principles of marketing professional services.
- Target your services to a segment of your community.
- Explore efficient methods to inform potential clients about your services.

INTRODUCTION

This chapter will discuss marketing concepts as they relate to professional services. An organized marketing plan will reveal two important things about your clients: what they want and what they will pay for your services. Healthcare marketing often misses its target by focusing on end users of services rather than individuals who may make purchasing decisions. A marketing plan identifies who makes purchase decisions about the types of services you will offer and then prepares information directed toward those individuals. This chapter will also identify specific methods of informing clients about your services.

MARKETING DEFINED

Marketing begins with gathering information about what individuals and groups want and need, then developing a program to meet those desires, next informing people that an opportunity exists, and finally allowing exchanges of value between provider and consumer (Kotler, Hayes & Bloom, 2002). The value of your practice to potential clients, while complex, basically comes down to what a client is willing to pay for what he wants. While developing plans for a community practice, you need to constantly compare services you want to offer with clients' actual wants and needs for those services. You also need to consider how you will use marketing to provide convincing information about the value of your services. Questions that need to be asked to develop a successful practice include:

- Who would be interested in the services I plan to offer?
- How much are clients willing and able to pay for these services?
- How will time considerations, such as frequency and duration, affect services?
- How will location of the practice determine its success?
- What specific outcomes can be expected from services provided?

A market analysis that begins with answers to these questions clarifies marketing as a process of consumer choice, which ultimately determines the success or failure of any service or product offered.

Marketing is sometimes confused with advertising and sales. While these functions are a part of the marketing process and are concerned with delivering your message about the program you offer, they emerge from market analysis. Market analysis occurs in tandem with developing a plan and an evaluation for your practice. These are not separate and sequential processes, but rather interrelated activities that will help bring about a program that is needed by the community and preferred over competing service options.

MARKET ANALYSIS

A market is a group of people or organizations, singled out from the entire community, likely to be interested in the services you plan to provide. You will need to learn about your potential clients through a process of research using both quantitative and qualitative methods of data collection and analysis. Clients' decisions to purchase are based on multiple aspects of a product or service including cost, location of delivery, promotion, perceived efficacy, and delivery method. Kotler, Hayes, and Bloom (2002) state that marketing professional services is challenging because the services cannot be separated from the professional who provides them.

Consumers make most major purchase decisions based on the product's purpose and cost. For example, most consumers in need of a car for personal transportation consider that new car to be a major purchase. They spend time comparing cars' features important to them or their family, and shop at various car dealerships before making a purchase. Car manufacturers and dealers invest in market analysis to determine what consumers want or need and what they are willing to pay. They then design and stock cars and develop advertising messages to target consumer preferences. Consumers will negotiate with a car dealer on price and features, and may delay a purchase if they cannot get what they want at the price they want to pay. When the auto industry does not produce what consumers desire at the price they are willing to pay, cars do not sell and businesses associated with the auto industry begin to fail.

Health care is unlike most consumer products. When someone needs healthcare services, there may be very limited resources in the community to choose from and little or no time to shop. Someone needing health care may find it difficult to identify what is needed and to differentiate among various types of service providers. In some cases, third-party payers make purchase decisions for their customers. Insurance providers decide which services they will pay for and specify who may deliver those services. If insurance companies refuse to pay for services, a client may be unwilling or unable to pay for services they may not understand or value. Healthcare providers deliver services based on their education, skill, and sometimes on what is reimbursable by insurance. They may, however, have little appreciation of clients' understanding regarding their need for services. Clients are likely to choose services based on factors unrelated to professional qualifications of the provider, especially if third-party reimbursement is not involved. A client's perception of service value and quality includes a provider's reliability, response to client needs, assurance that benefits will exceed costs, empathy, and caring. Clients also attach value to appearances, particularly of space, people, and written materials (Kotler, Hayes & Bloom, 2002).

The challenge to professional service providers is to integrate best practice with clients' perceptions of quality. This may best be accomplished through client centered care (Law & MacDermid, 2008). Successful community practice relies on client satisfaction, and development of a relationship results in repeated use of services or referral of others to your services.

Location

In community practice your market is probably going to be bounded by the location in which services are to be provided. This may include the entire community or only a segment of the community. Demographic data such as age, economic status, cultural preferences, and prevalence of the problems you intend to address—within a location specified by city, county, school district, or zip code—provides quantitative information to define your market. Depending upon the size of your community, you may choose to serve a large geographic area or focus on a smaller target area. Therapists who provide home based services often prefer to treat clients close to their homes to minimize driving time and travel cost. If, from observation and intuition, you identify a specific segment of the market—such as aging adults or young families—and believe it more likely than the general population to utilize your services, you will target your program to these people (Pakroo, 2008; Kotler, Hayes & Bloom, 2002). For example, if you want to direct services to children with a diagnosis of autism spectrum disorder (ASD) you would want to know the prevalence of this condition in the general population by age group, as well as the ages of children living in your community, to have some estimate of how many children may be potential clients. A suburban area with neighborhoods composed of young families is a likely target market for your services. If, on the other hand, you live in a rural community inhabited primarily by older adults and few children, this environment would be unlikely to generate the number of children you would need to make a pediatric practice financially sustainable. Such an environment could, however, provide opportunities for services targeted to aging adults.

It would be useful to know what type of public support, if any, exists for the problems you want to address in your practice. This will help you to determine whether there are public or private funds available for your services. Are you offering services that would enhance quality of life for many in the community? Is there is an economic advantage to addressing the problem? An example of an economic advantage would be reduced absenteeism for workers or their families needing rehabilitation services if those services are offered close to the work site. Services that contribute to community life are more likely to have the support of local employers or politicians, who may be able to influence your success by advocating for payment for your services.

Services

After identifying your target market, you need to further refine your understanding of what clients desire. Given the fact that potential clients of healthcare services may not understand differences among service providers, you want to determine how much your potential clients know about the services you provide. The best way to find out if the targeted market understands your services is to talk to them (Kotler, Hayes & Bloom, 2002). If people in your community or target market do not know about occupational therapy, or if they seem uncertain about whether or not your services would be beneficial, you want to educate them about your profession, the options that exist for services that you provide, and evidence that supports efficacy of these services (Phillips & Raspberry, 2008). You can collect data about need for services, and educate people in the community about occupational therapy, by meeting with groups or individuals to share information. You could also collect data about potential demand for your services by distributing a survey targeted to people who might use your services. For example, if you are thinking about offering aging-in-place home evaluations or driving assessments, you might develop a survey inquiring about needs for either for these services to be distributed through senior centers or in neighborhoods of older residents.

While you collect data about what clients might want or need, you may want to further explore what would attract clients to your practice. Convenience—including close proximity to home or work and hours that accommodate lifestyle—frequently motivates people to seek services.

Cost Considerations in Marketing

Cost for services is a significant factor for potential clients. Some clients seek healthcare services only if they are covered by insurance; others are willing to pay directly for services, but may have a cost threshold they cannot exceed. In making your decision about methods of payment for your services, you are segmenting your potential market into those clients who prefer the payment method(s) you have chosen. Other important considerations that might direct a person to your services are quality of life factors such as a desire to decrease pain, increase function, decrease feelings of guilt or sadness, decrease sense of burden, or increase optimism. Although these factors may not have a monetary cost associated with them, clients may place a high value on enhancing quality of life.

Time Considerations in Marketing

Community practice will likely depend upon new clients for sustainability. Healthcare services are limited in frequency and duration by third-party payers and therefore cannot be provided indefinitely to a client. If services are not paid for by insurance, there are still limits on how much most clients can pay for services. Healthcare services gain support from clients because they remedy clients' problems and eliminate the need for further services. Although some community practices maintain clients for long periods of time, most clients are relatively short term and their satisfaction with outcomes can become recommendations to others to use your services when a need arises. Personal recommendation is a powerful marketing tool and can help determine whether your program will succeed or not. Since you undoubtedly have limited resources, you will need information from market analysis to focus your marketing activities on those most likely to become your clients (Silverstein, 2006).

ASSESSING THE COMPETITION

Once you have determined that a population needing your services exists, you need to investigate programs or services similar to yours that are already active in your community. Competition can be a good thing since it keeps programs striving to deliver services preferred by consumers. For example, many communities now offer quite a good selection of coffee shops because when one coffee shop opens for business in a community the demand for specialty coffee increases and soon more coffee shops open in response to the first establishment. Competition continues as increasingly unique environments develop where customers can consume increasingly exotic coffee drinks. The trend to make a coffee shop a destination for more than just a quick beverage further increases demand for coffee shops; clients may choose to purchase coffee based on ambiance of the environment. As long as a need or desire for service exists, additional competitors increase demand for the service and keep the quality of services high. The same principle also applies to professional services. Establishing an appealing environment may differentiate your services from those of competitors, while at the same time increasing demand for services for both your own and your competitors' practices.

If a practice similar to what you want to offer exists, find out as much as possible about its activities, professional services, and environment. Visit competitors and talk to their clients to find out what they like about the services. Some things that attract clients are price, convenient location, and hours of operation. Perhaps you can address some weaknesses of the competition by providing a more convenient location or hours that accommodate working parents. Chapter 8 described Strength, Weakness, Opportunity, and Threat (SWOT) analysis as a process to compare your strengths, weaknesses, opportunities, and threats from competitors. You want to use your strengths and your competitors' weaknesses as described by clients to create opportunities for your practice. What are the strengths of existing programs? In what areas are they unable to satisfy consumer desires? If you cannot improve on the offerings available, it probably is not worthwhile to develop your practice in the same area. You might consider planning your services to be complementary to the competition, which will benefit your community and strengthen your relationship with your colleagues as you refer clients to each other. According to game theory, if you put your competitor out of business by offering your services at a lower cost or through another client enticement, your community loses the benefit of having both practices in competition with each other. Competition keeps prices affordable to clients and raises expectations for quality service. Given that there are finite supplies of professional providers in any area, there are times you may want to work collaboratively with your competitors for the good of the community. Appreciating good competition is better than seeking to put it out of business.

Analysis of resources available for your practice is a consideration in your marketing strategies. Are there adequate skilled personnel for you to hire if you plan to expand your practice in the future? Most likely you know the availability of such people in your community; if not, you can contact your state professional organization for the distributions of credentialed personnel in your area. You will benefit from having contact with these professional resources and making your practice an attractive alternative for collaboration or future employment. You may want to talk with students and educators, or members of community organizations, who may be able to serve as volunteers, future employees, or referrals for your practice.

Some Web sites provide resources that may help in analyzing the competition and developing a marketing plan. The Small Business Association, for example, offers suggestions on how to learn more about competitors and prepare marketing plans.

MARKETING TO THOSE WHO MAKE PURCHASING DECISIONS

Peters (2005) provides some valuable information for therapists who are considering developing a community practice. He points out that women make 80% of the decisions regarding health care and are responsible for two-thirds of healthcare spending, yet most healthcare marketing activities are designed to appeal to men (Peters, 2005). Dychtwald and Flowers (1990) stated that older adults controlled 70% of all wealth in the country and spend many billions of dollars on health care. In 2008, the American Association of Retired Persons (AARP) reported that people older than 55 own 77% of all financial assets in the United States, and account for 45% of consumer spending, or $2.1 trillion a year. A report by the U.S. Census Bureau reveals that in the period from 2005 to 2007, 80% of adults 65 years and older had a mean average income of $70,000 and 80% of the population was at, or 150% above, the poverty level. Even in challenging economic times most aging adults are able to continue purchasing services that help them maintain independence. As the aging adult population increases, they may demand improved funding for healthcare services directed toward aging in place. Your practice planning and marketing planning can benefit from your knowledge that aging adults have money to spend, are not planning to surrender to an inactive aging process, and are accustomed to being well served. If you examine your service ideas, most likely you will identify that women or aging adults will be making the decisions about your services for a family member or for themselves. Consider designing your marketing messages to appeal to their needs and desires.

Promotion to Women

What do we know about women that can influence our marketing strategies to this segment of the population? They want to connect on a personal level with service providers; they have a sense of responsibility for those in their care; and they think from a collective rather than an individual perspective. Generally, women enjoy talking and emotionally sharing with other women. Most women are experts at multitasking—almost a necessity of modern lifestyle. They enjoy being with others and respond more positively to narratives or storytelling rather than to charts and tables of data (Peters, 2005). Knowing this can help you understand that telling stories illustrating the benefits of your services will have an impact on women making healthcare decisions. You need look no further than women's magazines to see the impact of emotionally laden stories on influencing women's decisions. Stories connect readers to a situation while at the same time compelling them to act. You will want to develop stories about potential clients that present factual information in the style of fiction. If you are not sure how to do this, read some examples of human interest stories in magazines or newspapers and model your writing after these examples. Even if you have written stories in the past, many years of professional writing, which minimizes emotion and maximizes facts, may make this challenging. Your appeal to women decision makers is also more compelling when it is delivered through personal contact with someone with similar experiences. That is why word-of-mouth advertising is so effective when women are your clients.

Promotion to Aging Adults

In offering a community service to aging adults, you will have an advantage if you keep in mind that generally this market segment likes to retain control of their lives and plans to remain active into old age. Much advertising to aging adults has been targeted to their children and not infrequently portrays the parent-child relationship in reverse, with an adult child caring and making decisions for an aging parent. These advertisements often feature an unflattering portrayal of an elderly person who has difficulty with physical activities and typically appears confused or depressed. You can see that such portrayals would be insulting to a generation of people who plan to stay active and in charge, and who have the resources to remain independent even if they physically can no longer manage this. An alternative portrayal of aging is offered in the pages of magazines directed at the aging population, such as *AARP, The Magazine*, in which feature articles and advertising show older adults engaged in active lifestyles.

Aging adults will continue to work and play as they choose, and most of them intend to continue to drive even as their physical abilities may diminish. Offering services to these clients in communities where affluent aging adults live will enable them to make choices and pay for those choices. Access to demographic information about age and income will substantially assist you in developing and marketing your community practice to target these aging adults. Your opportunity to have a successful community practice lies in providing aging adults with options to make their lives easier and more satisfying.

HOW TO LET THEM KNOW YOU EXIST

At the beginning of this chapter, we specified that marketing is not advertising, and yet informing clients that you have something to exchange with them is part of marketing. In advertising your services, you will need to distribute appropriate information to potential clients about services you offer that can meet some of their needs or desires. You will want to establish a unique identity, a brand, for your practice. Branding is the term used to describe how your services are differentiated from those of other service providers (Silverstein, 2006). Branding your practice will tell clients who you are, why you are engaged in providing your services, and how you are special and better than other service providers (Peters, 2005). As you develop a brand for your business, think about how your services will make a difference in people's lives and why clients might choose what you offer over services offered by your competitors.

Continue your marketing plan by working out a few branding statements describing how your practice offers unique services that illustrate how much you care about your clients and your work. The brand you have chosen may point you toward a logo or slogan for your practice that you will use in marketing and that current and future clients associate with your excellent services (Phillips & Raspberry, 2008). Design your logo around your brand. For example, if your practice serves children, you might incorporate a toy, such as a teddy bear or blocks, into your logo. If you plan to offer driving assessments, consider using a steering wheel as part of your logo.

If you have worked with potential clients, educating them about your profession and your services throughout your market analysis and program planning processes, your potential clients will know about your program even before you open your doors. Because you sought their opinions while developing the program, they are likely to expect that you listened to them and incorporated their preferences into the services you offer. Consequently, some of your work is already done; these clients may simply be waiting for you to begin your community practice.

You may have other potential clients you will want to reach with a message about your services. In addition to clients or caregivers of clients, you will want to inform people who may become potential referral sources. Other providers of health or rehabilitative services are good targets for an informative message about your practice. These include physicians, social workers, other therapists, teachers, and third-party payers who will influence use of your services. Each of these groups of influential people may have a different concern in referring their clients to your practice. You need to consider different messages for each. Physicians may respond best to a written document that cites efficacy studies of services you will offer; they may prefer to have statistics as part of this presentation. Teachers want to know how your services would enhance a child's learning or reduce behavior problems in the classroom. You might consider that the majority of teachers are women, and appeal to women's preferences for storytelling as part of a marketing message (Peters, 2005). Third-party payers are interested in saving money, so a message about return on investment would be relevant to their needs. You might want to present information focusing on outcome studies that show how benefits outweigh costs of treatment.

MARKETING MEDIA

You may have available a variety of different media to deliver the message about benefits of your practice to your targeted audiences. As you select the best medium for your message, consider how much it will cost you to develop and deliver your message, and how potential clients are likely to seek information about services when a need arises. Advertising costs can be high, and many small businesses and private practices may be unable to pay consultants to develop print or broadcast media. Although advertising in phone books or in local newspapers may be beneficial, short, factual, and personalized letters to other healthcare or education providers may be a good way for them to learn about your practice and inform others of your services. Make sure your letter tells how you are uniquely qualified to provide services. Having special credentials for treatment methods, or holding advanced degrees, may provide you with an edge over your competitors. In your letter, state that you will phone the recipient to answer any questions he or she might have or to provide additional information about your qualifications or your services. Always follow up as promised; this will demonstrate that you are reliable and take your business responsibilities seriously. If possible, schedule a visit to potential referral sources to tell them about your practice and your services. Plan a convincing oral presentation, and prepare written materials to leave behind at the time of the visit. These materials must be well written and concise; claims should be supported by evidence.

One cost-effective method to introduce potential women clients to your services is to bring them together for a special event. This could be an open house or a support group meeting that you host at your work location. Bringing your current clients together with potential clients allows word-of-mouth advertising to promote your services. Consider phoning service organizations, parent groups, senior citizen clubs, or any other organization that would like to have a speaker for one of their meetings. Such a setting would provide an ideal opportunity for you to talk about your practice, describe the community need you would like to address with your services, and tell some stories about how you got started. You could also describe your professional background and some of your clients' successes. Perhaps a client would join you in talking to others about his experience with your services; it would be more powerful to have a client tell his story than for you to talk generically about what you provide. If you have the opportunity, you could offer to provide a short presentation to other service providers describing the latest research or treatment techniques offered for clients of mutual interest. Follow up with a description of how you incorporate these treatment approaches into the services you provide.

You also might want to write a special-interest story to be published in the local newspaper or as a short article in a newsletter that is sent to potential clients. Many local newspapers welcome stories of interest to their subscribers, and this becomes free advertising for your practice. If you are offering a community service that is unique and makes a significant contribution to quality of life for people living in your community, news media are likely to be interested in reporting about your practice as a public service. You might want to participate in local events such as a health fair in order to let your community know of the services you are providing through your practice.

Brochures you develop for clients could be posted in locations they are likely to visit. You will need permission to leave your brochures at these locations, but this may be an effective method to let others know of your services. In order to gain the attention of readers, the brochure should use noticeable and attractive colors or graphics. You will want to highlight your service with a catchy statement or slogan regarding its potential benefits. Follow with a brief narrative of your services to expand clients' understanding of what you offer. Techniques that catch people's attention are the use of bullet points, photos, and graphics. Make sure you have permission to use photos of people, whether they are clients, friends, or your own children. Use action-oriented photographs or illustrations, and if possible print your brochure in color to better attract people's attention. If you use a logo, make sure it is prominent on your brochure and include all of your contact information so that if someone is interested in your services they can get in touch with you easily.

The internet provides an opportunity to get information to potential clients at reasonable cost, but there are advantages and disadvantages to using this medium to inform clients of your community practice. Although developing a Web site to reach your potential clients may seem like a good idea, keep in mind that while Web sites reach many people, some of those people may not be living in your community. Olson and Dillon (2006) state that consumers are increasingly using the internet for information about health concerns and treatment options, but not everyone has access to the internet—particularly people who are economically disadvantaged or aging. Developing a Web site can be expensive if you hire someone to design your site, and monthly maintenance costs vary from reasonable to very expensive for most small businesses (Calandra, 2004). You could develop the site yourself, but unless it looks professional, it may not help attract clients to your practice. On the other hand, if your competitors are using a Web site, you may want to develop a site for your practice to educate clients and differentiate your services from others (Calandra, 2004; Phillips & Raspberry, 2008).

Details about developing a Web site for your business are beyond the scope of this book but are available in books devoted to the topic. Some considerations, however, apply whether you are developing a Web site or using other print media for advertising. In developing a Web site you will need to create an address and design content for your site. Web addresses should connect potential clients to your practice; therefore you will want to incorporate something easy to remember about your practice. Consider using the name of your practice while adding a word descriptive of your work.

Your address needs to be unique and not currently in use by someone else. Once you have found a Web address that meets these criteria you can register your address so others cannot use it.

The contents of your Web page need to be well organized, easy to read, and attractive to potential clients. Include your logo and name followed by the most important points about your practice. This is similar to information you would include on a brochure, but with a Web site, you can continuously add and update materials. Add links to relevant chat rooms or other Web sites providing more information about clinical conditions, occupational therapy services, and any other information that your clients or their families might find helpful. A Web site requires regular maintenance to update information and keep the site fresh and relevant to clients.

In branding your practice you developed an image that sets you apart from competitors. Just as consumers prefer a certain brand when purchasing sporting equipment or food products because they are consistently satisfying, you want consumers in your community to value your services and look for your brand. Use your name and logo in all advertising so that potential clients look for these in choosing services. Your business card is part of your brand. Design it to include your logo and contact information. Business cards can be developed on your computer or you can have them designed at office supply stores. You can print cards by the sheet in an office supply store or order and print 100 or more. Before you print the first card, be sure that all information is accurate and spelled correctly. It is a good idea to have someone else proofread your business card design before having cards mass produced. Some practices continue branding by having all employees dress in clothing that displays your business logo, a practice that can also become advertising of your services.

In order to maintain successful marketing strategies, and change or abandon those that are not working for you, you will want to know which of your strategies is most effective in attracting clients to your practice. Many of the marketing strategies identified in this chapter are free or minimal-cost, but when you use more costly methods, you want to be sure they are effective in attracting clients to your practice. One way to evaluate your marketing strategies is to ask new clients how they heard about your practice. If most clients are coming to you because they have been referred by other clients, then you know that word-of-mouth is your most effective marketing strategy. Even though you identify one marketing strategy as very effective in generating new clients, you should continue to develop and evaluate other methods to get information about your practice to potential clients.

Whichever strategies you use to attract customers, the goal is to keep them satisfied so that they utilize your services as needed and refer others to your practice. Keeping existing clients is easier than generating new ones. Peppers and Rogers (2008) state that doing the right thing for your clients will keep them loyal to you. Peters (2005) recommends that you maximize your value to your clients by fulfilling their dreams so that they want more of your services and want to share their experiences with others. These authors reflect the choice of developing a community practice to serve the needs of others and also to become successful in business. Marketing will help you achieve both goals. Brander (2008) suggests focusing on customer service while marketing in a weak economy, and using less costly means of getting your message to clients by text messaging, speaking to community groups, writing for local papers to show your expertise, and volunteering with groups that may yield future clients.

CHAPTER SUMMARY

This chapter has described marketing as a process of learning about your clients—their wants, needs, and willingness to pay for a service. Information about clients and the community environment in which you plan to practice is critical to your success, and this chapter has described examples of how to collect relevant information. Knowing who to market your services to will make your job easier. Women and aging adults have influence over healthcare choices and have resources to support services of benefit to their lifestyles. Targeting your marketing to these groups of potential clients will produce results through growth of your practice. We identified specific methods, focusing on free or low-cost options, to get the message about your services to potential clients. Choices available include personal contact, brochures, letters, Web sites, and community services.

LEARNING ACTIVITIES

These activities are designed to focus your attention on developing a message that attracts clients to your practice.

1. Knowing your client is necessary before you can determine how to appeal to his or her interest in using the services of your community practice.

   Write a description of the client who will benefit from your services. This client profile will focus on client needs and desires related to community participation and should include relevant characteristics such as age, socioeconomic status, disabilities, culture, and interests.

2. Identify additional stakeholders who are important to the success of your practice, such as caregivers or referral sources. Write a statement that describes what they want from your services.

3. How do you expect clients to learn about your new community practice? What message will they want to hear? What media may attract their attention?

   List each stakeholder group you want to inform about your community practice.

   Identify specific information that each group needs in order to decide to choose your service. Identify media that would appeal to each stakeholder group.

4. Prepare a list of media you will use to inform stakeholders of your practice, such as Web page, letter, or your participation in a community meeting. What are the costs to prepare or carry out each message about your practice? How many paying clients will you likely provide services to as the result of each method? Which method of marketing your services seems to be the most cost effective?

5. Prepare a sample letter that might be sent to a professional asking him or her to refer clients to your new community practice. Consider including evidence of best practice along with specific information about how clients will benefit from your services.

6. Write a story about a client who has benefited from your services. This can be fiction, but will be based on your knowledge of client needs, your professional expertise, and evidence of best practice. Develop your story with the intent of emotionally attracting potential clients to your practice.

7. Keeping in mind your clients, the services you will provide, and community culture, develop a logo and slogan that will assist in establishing a brand for your community practice.

References

American Association of Retired Persons (AARP) (2008). Because we are powerful. *AARP Magazine, September/October*, 61.

Brander, J. (2008). Marketing in a weak economy. SCORE Podcast retrieved December 18, 2008 from http://www.sbtv.com/?segid=3356

Calandra, B. (2004). Caught in the web. *Fitness Business Pro, 20* (11) 38–41.

Dychtwald, K. & Flowers, J. (1990). *Age wave: How the most important trend of our time can change your future.* New York, NY: Bantam Books.

Kotler, P., Hayes, T. & Bloom, P.N. (2002). *Marketing professional services* (2nd ed.). NJ: Prentice Hall.

Law, M.C. & MacDermid, T. (2008). *Evidence-based rehabilitation: A guide to practice.* Thorofare, NJ: Slack.

Olson, A. & Dillon, B. (2006). Staying power: Convert website visitors to patients. *Marketing Health Services, 26* (2) 38–41.

Pakroo, P.H. (2008). *The small business start-up kit* (5th ed.). Berkeley, CA: Nolo.

Peppers, D. & Rogers, M. (2008). *Rules to break and rules to follow: How your business can beat the crisis of short-termism.* Hoboken NJ: John Wiley & Sons.

Phillips, H. & Raspberry, S. (2008). *Marketing without advertising: Easy ways to build a business your customers will love and recommend* (6th ed.). Berkeley, CA: Nolo.

Peters, T.C. (2005). *Re-imagine! Business excellence in a disruptive age.* London: Dorling Kindersley.

Silverstein, R. (2006). *The best secrets of great small businesses.* Naperville, IL: Resourcebook.

Solie-Johnson, K. (2005). *How to set up your own small business, Vol. 2.* Minneapolis, MN: American Institute of Small Business.

ELECTRONIC RESOURCES

Business stationery templates
www.VistaPrint.com.

Small Business Administration marketing ideas and suggestions
http://www.sba.gov/smallbusinessplanner/manage/marketandprice. Retrieved December 17, 2008.

U.S. Census Bureau
http://factfinder.census.gov. Retrieved December 18, 2008.

Chapter 11

Linking Evaluation with Planning, Financing, and Marketing Your Service

- Distinguish types of evaluation.
- Consider benefits of utilizing a logic model to evaluate your practice.
- Identify evaluation methods linking cost with outcomes.
- Utilize evaluation to provide useful information to sustain your program.

INTRODUCTION

This chapter will link evaluation to designing and implementing a community practice. Although evaluation is generally considered a process of appraisal to determine value of program outcomes, it is also a process to shape a developing practice. Designing a program evaluation should begin as soon as ideas are formulated for community practice, and continue throughout the development of program, financial, and marketing strategies. Evaluation data will inform each decision about practice, and contribute evidence of progress toward your community practice goals.

EVALUATION IS AN INTEGRATED FUNCTION OF PRACTICE

Politics of Evaluation

Evaluation serves many purposes throughout the life span of a community practice. Ideas for practice may be intuitive, but more often they are based on some quantitative or qualitative data you have accessed or generated that indicates a need for services. Evaluation may be considered a political process because you will have the potential to influence decision makers with the types of evidence you choose to use in support of your practice. Demographic data or information from surveys or focus groups can influence decisions about financial support for practice if you demonstrate that your services meet a community need and provide good value to potential clients and other stakeholders. Evaluation can also be the means to demonstrate publicly the positive impact of your services on your community. Evaluation provides a political legitimation of the efficacy of your services that may be difficult to achieve in any other way.

Decisions about what will be included or excluded from evaluation are political because these choices influence clients, potential lenders, and other stakeholders with an interest in your practice. Grembowski (2001) describes program evaluation as a process of accountability for healthcare services in an environment where there is concern about escalating costs, scarce resources, and evidence-based practice. Evaluation is conducted in a political context with a variety of competing interests. It applies techniques and methods of social science to provide informed judgments about a program's worth.

Evaluation to Support Practice Development

As you begin to consider options for community practice, evaluation informs you of needs that exist within your community—information you will utilize as you assess your potential for success. In surveying the landscape to discover a need for your practice, you gathered data to support your decision to go forward with your plans (Berk & Rossi, 1999). You projected costs associated with starting your practice and determined whether you had sufficient resources available or would require outside financing. Based on these data, you either proceeded to develop your practice or reconsidered your plans. As you entered the development phase of your practice, you used evaluation results to make decisions about clinical, financial, and marketing activities. Each major decision in developing community practice is preceded by collecting and analyzing data, and the results of analysis either move you forward or cause you to reconsider your plans.

In developing a practice plan, you reviewed professional journals for evidence of best practice and decided which services to provide based on evidence of efficacy. Standards for excellence gleaned from your literature review will become benchmarks for outcomes at various stages of your practice. The wonderful thing about program evaluation is that it requires you to collect data from the outset of planning and gives you an opportunity to modify your practice in response to these data. If you find that the evidence available about the type of practice you want to offer is insufficient for your population or environment, the data you collect may point you to another more effective practice approach. You can do this as soon as you discover a discrepancy between your desires and your clients' needs and not wait until the end of an evaluation cycle to correct your service delivery. By waiting, you could lose your clients and your practice. In the development phase of practice, you also will make decisions about hiring additional personnel, locating your practice, and handling financing. All of these decisions will be better informed if you have established criteria for what you desire, as well as obtained data that show how well you are performing these functions. If you plan to provide services that require specialized clinical skills, you will use these criteria in hiring decisions. The outcomes of evaluation can provide reassurance that your decisions have been based on the best available evidence and that you are maximizing your potential for success.

Evaluation to Support Economic Development

Evaluation criteria for financing your practice are especially important to your success. You will need to put together budgets and financial plans if you seek external funding, and financiers may require you to have a program evaluation in place before they will consider whether or not to give you the money you need to start your practice. Financiers will be concerned about whether you have thought through revenue production to cover your costs and whether your service will generate outcomes that result in future cost savings (Drummond, O'Brien, Stoddart & Torrance, 1999). The quantitative data you project for costs and revenue become monetary objectives to be compared with your actual expenses and income each month. As time elapses, you can build graphs representing financial performance of your practice. Time series graphs may offer reassurance during the early months, when it is difficult to generate income that exceeds expenses, that your practice has established a trend toward profitability.

Evaluation to Support Marketing Decisions

Marketing decisions benefit from a well conceived evaluation that reveals the effectiveness of methods you use to get information about your practice to clients. Although your data support the need for your services, and thus inform your practice development plan, deciding which types of message and media will provide the best outcomes for your practice requires evaluation. You may know what type of advertising has worked well in your community for similar services and plan to use the same approach as you begin your practice. It would be better, however, to design an evaluation process to assure yourself that this is an effective approach to gaining your share of the clients available in your community. If a specific marketing activity, such as a brochure, helped you attract clients you expect to serve, you can evaluate the actual number of clients who report they found your practice from your brochure. This helps you determine if you are using the correct media and message to attract the clients your practice needs to survive.

Types of Evaluation

Issel (2004) identifies types of evaluation corresponding to different stages in the life cycle of a community health program. This approach supports the need to develop program evaluation as you first explore the feasibility of starting a new community practice.

- Evaluating *community needs* prior to beginning practice informs program planning.
- As a program begins operation, *process evaluation* monitors your actions to see if you are sticking to your plan.
- *Outcomes evaluation* reflects whether or not your services are making a difference in your community.
- *Efficiency evaluation* correlates your costs with outcomes.
- *Meta evaluation* compares your outcomes over time, as well as your outcomes with those of other programs similar to your practice.

You will want to consider using each of these types of evaluation to provide evidence of the merit and worth of your practice to your community.

WHO WILL EVALUATE YOUR PROGRAM? WHAT SKILLS ARE NEEDED?

The response to the first question may seem obvious. It will be you. After all, you may be starting a very small practice as a sole practitioner, and not have financial resources to hire an external evaluator. The answer to the second question, however, may complicate your answer to the first question. You may not have the skills needed to be an effective evaluator. If you conduct your own evaluation you will need to gather data about your efficacy as service provider, community preferences for types of service, and standards of excellence in clinical practice and management. This information is needed to make decisions and institute program changes that will benefit your clients and your practice. The obvious advantage of being your own evaluator is minimizing cost, but another advantage is that you can alter your evaluation design rapidly if your original plan is ineffective in providing the information you need to make decisions. You are the person best able to understand your practice, including where to look for data you need to be credible to others (Owen, 2007).

Carman (2007) identifies questions that might be asked in designing evaluations for community-based organizations:

- What types of activities are to be used for evaluation? If data results are subjected to external audits, used for performance reviews of staff, or to meet accreditation standards, data must be adequate to meet these needs.
- What types of data are to be collected? Demographic data usually is collected, but you will also want anecdotal information about the program's ability to satisfy client needs, as well as financial data to report to funders and for tax purposes.
- How will data be collected? Both quantitative and qualitative methods will be used including surveys, interviews, focus groups, and performance tests.
- Who is responsible for conducting the evaluation? Most community program evaluations are conducted by management staff of those programs.
- What is the funding source for the evaluation? Community programs either absorb the cost of evaluation or allocate money within the budget for this function.

If you have previous experience developing and implementing an evaluation, perhaps in a clinical role, you may have the skills needed to be your own evaluator. Most occupational therapy clinical program evaluations designed for use by institutions focus on technical aspects of therapy interventions that are observable and measurable and serve the purpose of the organization for which they are designed. Although data generated by this type of evaluation is important to the overall function of the organization, it may not adequately portray the value of occupational therapy service, and likely does not include much of the data that will be critical to your practice's survival.

If you are planning to be your own evaluator, therefore, you will want to have good research design skills in order to include both quantitative and qualitative methods of data collection and analysis. You will need to know what types of data are relevant to answering specific questions and solving problems encountered in planning and implementing practice. You will then choose evaluation methods that provide results for defensible decisions. Effective negotiation and communication skills can help you use your evaluation results for the benefit of your practice (Owen, 2007).

The American Evaluation Association (2004) publishes guiding principles for evaluators that further outline the competencies and ethical requirements for evaluators. Books about evaluation methods are among the numerous resources that might be helpful in developing an evaluation for your practice. You may want to consider enrolling in a continuing education course that teaches theory and practical applications of program evaluation. If you do not have skills needed to develop and implement an evaluation, you may hire a consultant to help you with this process. Davidson (2005) suggests that program evaluation designed and implemented for accountability should utilize an independent evaluator who is not invested in its activities. Carman (2007) says that by using an internal evaluator, community-based programs miss an opportunity to collect valuable data to help them improve their services. Considering the advantages and disadvantages of using an internal versus an external evaluator can help you make the best decision about how to accomplish this process.

LOGIC MODEL EVALUATION

All evaluation begins with a plan. Although there are different approaches to planning evaluation, use of a logic model may be helpful in developing evaluation for your practice. A logic model describes how a program will operate in a specific environment to solve identified problems (McLaughlin & Jordan, 2004). Morell (2005) says that a logic model of evaluation identifies the process variables and outcomes that you want to measure, the comparisons that you want to make, and causal chains expected if a program is operating as planned.

The first step in developing a logic model or any other type of evaluation is to identify stakeholders, who are defined as any person with an interest in your program. Stakeholders include clients, service providers, payers, related agencies, or referral sources. These individuals or groups of people with a common concern can each provide you with their expectations of your community practice. As you define practice context and identify community problems, information from stakeholders will help you determine whether your plans for service match the desires of residents in your community. Next, identify cause-and-effect linkages in which each individual or collective need is linked to a solution through your services. Clarify where community problems may be addressed by other services in addition to your own. If you plan to collaborate with others, establish responsibility for outcomes (McLaughlin & Jordan, 2004).

An example of a very simple logic model for a practice addressing a need to minimize cost associated with injured workers shows relationships among resources, activities, products, clients, and outcomes. The intent of the model is to find cause-and-effect linkages, which have a significant impact on the value of this service. Process variables are resources and activities that create products or services for clients that contribute to desired outcomes. The diagram shows that resources applied in work environments to screen for potential injuries enhance quality of life for workers in the community. Cost savings to employers result from evaluation and intervention services to employees that improve their function, enabling them to return to work following an injury.

As you define components of the logic model for your practice, understand how any changes in the environment may influence your practice. To design a logic model for your practice, start with a large sheet of paper and

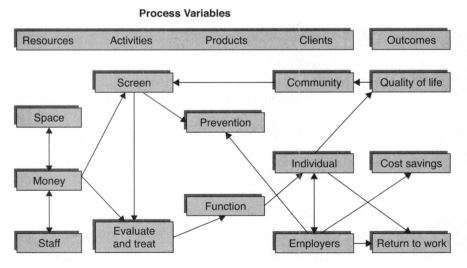

Figure 11–1 An example of logic model evaluation

begin diagramming a flow chart of process variables and desired outcomes. As you identify resources available for your practice and the activities you plan to provide, you establish the linkages between needs and expected outcomes. This will be an iterative process and you may miss components and linkages at first, but you can always add them as you go along. Describe all elements of how your service will work for you and for your clients. Consider any possible occurrences that might result in unexpected outcomes for your practice, both client outcomes as well as your business outcomes. Are there any logical partnerships that you could form to improve the outcomes of your services for clients or for your business? Continually ask yourself questions about why you are planning specific actions and search for alternatives that might give a different outcome. As you diagram your model of flow and linkages on paper, discuss it with stakeholders and benefit from their reflections on your work. Evaluation is all about making changes that work for you and for your clients. In a constantly changing environment you will need to be flexible and willing to change to survive (Peters, 2005).

Elliott, O'Neal, and Velde (2001) used chaos theory to better understand threats and opportunities in occupational therapy community practice. They wrote that community practice requires unpredictable interactions that have unanticipated results. In chaos theory there is constant interaction among elements of the environment that have potential to be either positive in creating new opportunities or, conversely, lead to disintegration of a program. The problem is that there is no way to predict and control outcomes of a complex open system such as a community practice. There are benefits, however, in attempting to identify potential changes in the environment that could be either beneficial or disastrous, in hopes of taking advantage of opportunity and mitigating disaster (Elliot, O'Neal & Velde, 2001). Including chaos theory in developing a logic model requires you to stretch beyond your current comfort level with predictable events and consider what environmental changes are possible in a complex environment. An example is economic change, which may have a profound effect on community practice and which has been difficult to predict. Keep abreast of things happening in your community and consider how any change could affect your practice.

Evaluation Components

Once your logic model is completed, you will be able to identify evaluation components and measurement points where data collection and analysis are needed.

Some areas you probably want to evaluate are productivity and efficiency. Although these terms have developed a negative connotation as organizations strive to increase revenue, both concepts are very important to a community practice. You will need to determine how much revenue you need to produce in order to stay in business, cover your expenses, and make a profit. Service quality or client satisfaction is important to evaluate, since this will also result in the success or failure of your community practice. Outcomes of service related to goal attainment are essential if you are obtaining third-party payment for your services. Consider data collection as an opportunity to discover how well you are performing relative to your mission and goals, and to learn the best approach for improving client satisfaction or expanding your services.

Methods of Data Collection

You will want to use both qualitative and quantitative methods of data collection. You cannot avoid quantitative activities when you are operating your own practice, because numbers are powerful representations of your success in meeting client expectations and your own monetary goals. On the other hand, qualitative data can have political implications since they involve stakeholders' determination of the value and ultimate success of your practice.

Qualitative data allow stakeholders' voices to be heard and empower clients. Sullins (2003) described an empowerment model of evaluation in which consumers and providers at a community mental health center collaboratively designed and implemented an evaluation in which they learned from each other how to improve their program. Preskill, Zuckerman, and Matthews (2003) demonstrated client and service provider collaboration through information exchange to improve service delivery in a cancer screening program. When you are in private practice, client satisfaction is likely the most important factor contributing to your success; listening to present and future clients becomes an essential component of your evaluation.

Trust in Evaluation Methods

Whatever methods you chose for data collection, they must be valid and reliable as well as meaningful to decision makers who will use the results. When you choose data collection methods, ask if the resulting data provides useful information needed by stakeholders to make beneficial decisions. Data should be balanced to include all stakeholders and provide a comprehensive picture of performance for your service. Ideally you will choose to include measures that allow comparison with other service options, or with benchmarks that you have established for your service.

When selecting your methods of data collection, you also need to be practical and consider how data will be collected and who will collect it. The challenge for an internal evaluator is to make time for this activity. In community practice, time is money and any time you spend on data collection will detract from time spent providing service. Without the benefit of evaluation, however, you will not have data to support your business decisions, which can also be costly. This time and money trade-off may lead you to hire an external evaluator, or to pay someone to collect and analyze data while you retain control of the evaluation design and process.

Data Analysis

After data is collected, it must be analyzed. Quantitative data is subjected to statistical analysis; qualitative data must be analyzed and categorized in such a way as to offer results useful to stakeholders. Statistical analysis need not be difficult. Often, descriptive or correlative analysis best serves the program evaluator and these are easily done with a computer program. Qualitative data analysis, although more labor- and time-intensive, may prove valuable in uncovering unanticipated outcomes. Qualitative data can reveal why your service is preferred over another service or can identify opportunities for offering additional services in your community (Heard, Greaves & Doe, 2001; Meyers, 1989). Miles and Huberman (1994) illustrate methods of analyzing qualitative data including meta-matrices, causal diagrams, and clustering to create visual displays of data that can be highly effective in reporting results of program evaluation. Among these methods, cause-and-effect diagrams illustrate the effectiveness of community practice by directly linking positive client outcomes with your service. Time series meta-matrices show changes made to your services over time and include feedback from clients or other stakeholders (Miles & Huberman, 1994).

Grembowski (2001) suggests that collecting both qualitative and quantitative sources of data for program evaluation enables you to triangulate and enhance the credibility of your results. Davidson (2005) recommends synthesizing qualitative and quantitative data into the overall evaluation of your program because both formative and summative results reveal strengths and areas for improvement of your service.

ECONOMIC EVALUATION

Economic evaluation may not be an immediate consideration when you are in the midst of planning community practice. There are, however, some very good reasons to include an economic component in your evaluation.

You are investing in your business and are concerned about success. If you have investors, they consider economic indicators of your success as return on their investment. Often in occupational therapy we look at outcomes of our services as future cost savings; that is, our services will prevent more costly healthcare or maintenance needs in the future. Economic evaluation methods are designed to assess economic impact and assist in healthcare decision making. There are four methods of economic analysis to consider including in your program evaluation: (1) cost-feasibility analysis; (2) cost-effectiveness analysis; (3) cost-benefit analysis; and (4) cost-utility analysis.

Cost-Feasibility Analysis

When you are in the planning stage, considering whether or not to go forward with your idea for community practice, you likely will be engaged in a process of cost-feasibility analysis. This process estimates the costs of practice alternatives to see if any can be considered for implementation based solely on cost or on your ability to financially support such a practice. You will need to identify all of the potential costs involved in starting and operating your practice, and then determine whether you can locate the financial resources necessary to implement your practice. If you plan to finance your own practice, a cost-feasibility analysis will allow you to see the total costs and determine whether you can afford them. If you are going to request a loan to get your practice started, you likewise will know if you qualify for a loan as large as you need, based on the budgeted cost and your credit rating. Cost-feasibility analysis allows you to determine at the outset whether you can afford to start the practice as planned; if not, you have an opportunity to abandon that particular practice plan (Levitt & McEwan, 2001).

Cost-Effectiveness Analysis

Cost-effectiveness analysis helps determine the best use of your resources. It aims to maximize the effectiveness of your resources in order to obtain the most value from your investment. With this process you select among different options for service delivery, such as client evaluation methods or interventions, and determine which gives the most efficient outcome. As you develop your community practice, you will have a finite amount of money to invest and will have to make choices. This resembles working with a household budget where the limited amount of money available means that choices must be made based on necessity and on what offers the greatest satisfaction. For example, you want to look good and wear attractive clothing, but must stay within your household budget. In this case, you have to choose whether to spend money on a few durable but more expensive clothing items or spend the same amount of money on a greater number of less expensive clothing items. You must ask yourself which option gives you the greatest satisfaction.

Grant providers use cost-effectiveness analysis to decide which projects they will fund. They review each grant proposal with an eye toward funding the proposals that most closely reflect their interests and meet their objectives. They evaluate alternative uses of their money and make a choice to fund the projects that offer the greatest return on their resources while forwarding their own agenda.

Cost-effectiveness analysis requires you to identify all of the costs associated with the options chosen and your desired outcome. In practice, you may decide that you want to provide services that increase your clients' mobility and independence. There are many different combinations of services you could provide that would result in the same positive outcome. For each possible service that results in the desired outcome, identify its associated costs and then compare the alternatives to select the least costly service or most profitable options. You will use this information to determine which services you will offer clients in your community.

The main disadvantage of this method is that you cannot compare cost-effectiveness ratios among alternatives that have different outcomes, nor can you make an overall determination of whether a program is worthwhile in an absolute sense. This method relies on combining cost data generated as you developed your budget with effectiveness data that is predetermined (evidence-based); it is relatively easy to perform and will lead to decisions that you can be comfortable with.

Cost-Benefit Analysis

Cost-benefit analysis evaluates alternatives according to their costs and outcomes when each is measured in monetary terms. Each service alternative is assessed on its own merits to see if it is worthwhile, with the objective being services that maximize revenue or minimize costs. The challenge with this method of economic analysis is that all costs and all benefits must be assigned monetary values. Some outcomes of health services are difficult to monetarily quantify. Cost-benefit analysis, however, allows comparisons among services with different outcomes (Levitt & McEwan, 2001). While this method is helpful in decision-making, it requires some accounting skills to assign monetary values to all variables. This may make it impractical for you to use as you make decisions about your community practice.

Cost-Utility Analysis

Cost-utility analysis evaluates and compares alternatives according to their costs and outcomes as valued by an individual or group. Utility is the satisfaction that individuals express for outcomes of services. After actual or potential clients establish utility, the calculation for cost-utility analysis is similar to cost-effectiveness analysis. An advantage of cost-utility analysis is that it allows individuals to express preferences for outcomes that include many different options for consideration. For example, a client could choose from among surgery, medication, or rehabilitation, with costs and outcomes evaluated for each alternative. The measure that is most often used when making these decisions is the quality adjusted life years (QALY) that can be achieved with each option. QALYs, which quantify health benefits of different treatment options, were developed from surveys in which patients expressed their preference for different health states (Levitt & McEwan, 2001). The QALY scale assigns a score between 0 and 1 for every health condition, with 0=death and 1=full health, in an effort to rationalize trade-offs between satisfying clients and the cost of service. This approach does not assess whether the treatment is worth the cost, only if it is more worthwhile than another treatment.

Cost-utility analysis is the process your potential clients will use as they decide whether your services are worth their cost. If they have other options available for use of their financial resources, they will weigh the value of cost and outcomes of your services against other options available to them. For example, if you offer services to children with special needs, a family may weigh the costs and the perceived benefits of your services against services available in public school. You need to consider options potential clients have available to them when you establish your marketing plans, set prices, and identify outcomes. Keep in mind that clients will be searching for good value for their money.

If you decide to include economic analysis in your evaluation, you need to figure out which one of these methods to use. Each method provides data to inform specific economic decisions. At different stages of developing your practice some methods will seem more logical than others. Difficulty assigning monetary costs and benefits could limit your choices of evaluation methods. Cost-feasibility analysis during the early decision-making phase of practice development could help you decide whether you can afford to continue. As you design your practice, cost-effectiveness analysis would offer useful information about your potential service offerings. Cost-utility analysis would be useful as you plan marketing activities to appeal to potential clients. You will already have cost information from development of your budget; choosing to include some form of economic analysis will assist with and substantiate decisions you make regarding your practice.

OUTCOMES OF EVALUATION

Authenticity of Results

As you complete your program evaluation design, you want to choose rigorous methods of data collection and analysis that will be accepted by stakeholders. Qualitative research has revealed standards of rigor with particular relevance to program evaluation. Guba and Lincoln (1989) identify authenticity criteria as essential components of qualitative evaluation. Stakeholders are empowered as both generators and users of collected and analyzed data. Tactical authenticity refers to the degree to which participants and other stakeholders are empowered to act through their contributions to the evaluation's focus and strategies. In designing evaluation of your practice, it is a good idea to include stakeholders in identifying what should be evaluated and how data should be collected. Certain stakeholders, such as those who provide financial support, may require that economic analysis be part of the evaluation. Other stakeholders, however, may be more interested in how outcomes of services will be determined.

Catalytic authenticity refers to action that has been stimulated by and facilitated by the evaluation process. You make changes in your practice and improve your program in response to data as it is being collected and analyzed. Educative authenticity means that stakeholders who participate in evaluation at any phase better understand how others may view services differently. In collecting qualitative data in your practice evaluation, you will share others' opinions about the services you provide. For example, funders of your practice may view services based solely on cost, while clients may view services based on changes in function or on satisfaction with providers. While these views may differ considerably, all are equally relevant in the evaluation process. Ontological authenticity is the extent to which each participant in the evaluation modifies his or her views as a result of learning from others. For example, third-party payers may change their process of reimbursement after being informed of the value of a service to clients as a result of evaluation. The purpose of authenticity criteria is to be certain that all stakeholders have their views and values fairly represented in the evaluation and are empowered to take actions as they learn from the data collection and reporting processes.

Intended and Unintended Outcomes

Evaluators appreciate that outcomes from program evaluation can be both intended and unintended. Morell (2005) identifies two types of unintended outcomes that may emerge from evaluation: the unforeseen and the unforeseeable.

Unforeseen consequences arise from inadequate understanding of the program and its intended outcomes. This requires the evaluator to enhance her understanding about the program and facilitate better collaboration and understanding of the program among stakeholders. Unforeseeable outcomes result from changes in the environment occurring throughout the period of evaluation. Unforeseeable consequences often provide opportunities for better practice. Kushner (2000) writes that there is no such thing as a stable state. Client and service providers come and go, competition arrives in the community, and treatment preferences change as a result of research. This resonates to chaos theory where one needs to constantly be open to possibilities for change and be flexible enough to take advantage of changes as they occur. Constant data collection, analysis, and environmental scanning will allow you to benefit from your evaluation as changes occur.

Knowledge Production

When unanticipated outcomes are discovered, this provides opportunity to reflect on your service and examine whether you have found something innovative that might contribute to more effective service delivery. You may discover that the treatment you selected to use in your practice, while based on best available evidence, is in fact not effective in your community practice. Investigating why this happens is also part of program evaluation. Conversely, discovering you are doing something innovative and experiencing surprisingly good results also merits further evaluation. Consider these outcomes an opportunity to collaborate with other providers or researchers to further explore these phenomena and build evidence of effective or efficient practice in the community.

PRESENTATION OF EVALUATION RESULTS

As you collect and analyze data throughout the process of developing and implementing your program, you will make changes in your practice to respond to client and other stakeholder needs and desires. At various points in your practice operations, and at the conclusion of an evaluation cycle, you will disseminate your results to stakeholders. Lawrence, Gullickson, and Toal (2007) state that evaluation outcomes are valued if they are presented in formats that are useful to each distinct stakeholder group. Berk and Rossi (1999) believe that evaluations provide information needed for decision making, but the results can be political and result in controversy and criticism. When evaluating your own practice, one of the critical voices should be your own, accompanied by data to help you make your practice better, more user friendly, or more lucrative.

Presentation of evaluation results may require several different formats to meet the needs of different stakeholders. A formal written report following specific guidelines, and likely focusing on outcomes and accounting activities, may be required by an organization that has contributed funds to your practice. You may want to prepare a written or an oral report for individuals who have referred clients to your practice, just to let them know the results of services you provided. Results of your evaluation may contain compelling statements suitable for use in future marketing materials.

When presenting results, you want to gain the attention of your audience. This may be accomplished by telling an emotional story of success that will get people's attention and evoke response. Results should be presented clearly so that they stimulate necessary improvements to the service and also exhibit its value to clients and stakeholders. As you prepare your report, you need to consider your message. What do you want remembered about your practice? What have you discovered through your evaluation and recommendations for improved service?

Kushner (2000) states that evaluation results persuade others of the value of your service if you present credible data derived from rigorous methods of data collection and analysis. With excellent results, you establish benchmarks for future delivery of your services and possibly those of your competitors. Being specific about how this excellence was achieved may provide a reference point for your practice. If, on the other hand, your results indicate that you have not achieved your goals or that your service has not met clients' expectations, consider these results an opportunity to change what you are doing. Utilizing information provided by clients not fully satisfied with your services can support necessary changes to improve your services. No service remains static. It changes constantly, and your evaluation process and results identify changes you will need to make to respond to a dynamic environment. Program evaluation empowers you to justify your expenses, boast about your services, or show how you are providing a cost-effective service.

CHAPTER SUMMARY

This chapter covered the basic information about developing, implementing, and reporting a program evaluation. The process of developing your program evaluation should run parallel with other activities you will need to undertake as you develop a community practice. Evaluation activities support decision making in pre-planning, program development, financing, and marketing community practice. Utilizing data generated by your evaluation activities on a regular basis will help you respond to changes that may be constantly occurring in your community.

LEARNING ACTIVITIES

Program evaluation provides information to be used in decision making about every aspect of starting and maintaining a community practice.

1. Inventory what skills and knowledge you have to develop and implement evaluation of your practice. Include your knowledge and experience designing and implementing quantitative and qualitative methods of research. Are you confident in your ability to know which method of research to use for each type of decision you will make, or problem you will solve, in designing and implementing your community practice?

    Identify resources are available to assist you in developing evaluation for your community practice.

2. Review your list of your community practice stakeholders. What specific interests do they have in your practice? What outcomes does each stakeholder group expect? What type of information is each stakeholder group likely to want from you to prove the worth or value of your practice?

3. Prepare a narrative of one client who will receive direct services from your practice. List the client's needs, interventions you will provide to meet those needs, and how you and the client will determine the effectiveness of your services. In addition to intervention outcomes, consider the total experience from the client's perspective.

4. List the decisions that you will need to make at each point in developing and operating your community practice. What specific information do you need to make each decision? What data will you need to collect and how will you collect this data? How will you analyze the data? How may interpretation of results modify each decision?

5. What changes in your practice environment might you anticipate over the next year? What evaluation mechanisms will you want to put in place to recognize and respond to these changes?

6. Use the logic model described in this chapter to identify resources, process variables, planned activities, and anticipated outcomes for your practice. Show linkages that exist and points at which you will collect and analyze data to better predict outcomes. What methods of data collection and analysis will you use?

7. How will you use evaluation results to influence stakeholders?

REFERENCES

American Evaluation Association (2004). Guiding principles for evaluators. Retrieved from http://www.eval.org.

Berk, R.A. & Rossi, P.H. (1999). *Thinking about program evaluation* (2nd ed.). Thousand Oaks, CA: Sage.

Carman, J.G. (2007). Evaluation practice among community-based organization: Research into reality. *American Journal of Research, 28* (1) 60–75.

Davidson, E.J. (2005). *Evaluation methodology basics: The nuts and bolts of sound evaluation.* Thousand Oaks, CA: Sage.

Drummond, M.F., O'Brien, B., Stoddart, G.L. & Torrance, G.W. (1999). *Methods for the economic evaluation of health care programmes* (2nd ed.). Oxford: Oxford University Press.

Elliott, S., O'Neal, S. & Velde, B.P. (2001). Using chaos theory to understand a community-built occupational therapy practice. *Occupational Therapy in Health Care, 13* (3/4) 101–111.

Grembowski, D. (2001). *The practice of health program evaluation.* Thousand Oaks, CA: Sage.

Guba, E.G. & Lincoln, Y.S. (1989). *Fourth generation evaluation.* Newbury Park, CA: Sage.

Heard, P., Greaves, M. & Doe, J. (2001). Living the process in psychiatric vocational assessment: A consumer outcome perspective. *Occupational Therapy in Mental Health, 17* (2) 21–34.

Issel, L.M. (2004). *Health program planning and evaluation: A practical, systematic approach for community health.* Boston, MA: Jones & Bartlett.

Kushner, S. (2000). *Personalizing evaluation.* Thousand Oaks, CA: Sage.

Lawrence, F., Gullickson, A. & Toal, S. (2007). Dissemination: Handmaiden to evaluation use. *American Journal of Evaluation, 28* (3) 275–289.

Levitt, M. & McEwan, P.J. (2001) *Cost-effectiveness analysis: Methods and applications* (2nd ed.). Thousand Oaks, CA: Sage.

McLaughlin, J.A. & Jordan, G.B. (2004). Using logic models. In J.S. Wholey, H.P Hatry & K.E. Newcomer (Eds.) *Handbook of practical program evaluation* (2nd ed.) (pp. 7–32). San Francisco, CA: Jossey Bass.

Meyers, S. (1989). Occupational therapy treatment of an adult woman with an eating disorder: One woman's experience. *Occupational Therapy in Mental Health, 9* (1) 33–47.

Miles M.B. & Huberman, A.M. (1994). *Qualitative data analysis* (2nd ed.). Thousand Oaks, CA: Sage.

Morell, J.A. (2005). Why are there unintended consequences of program action and what are the implications for doing evaluation? *American Journal of Evaluation, 26* (3) 444–465.

Owen, J.M. (2007). *Program evaluation: Forms and approaches* (3rd ed.). NY: Guilford Press.

Peters, T.C. (2005). *Re-imagine! Business excellence in a disruptive age.* London: Dorling Kindersley Ltd.

Preskill, H., Zuckerman, B. & Matthews, B. (2003). An exploratory study of process use: Findings and implications for future research. *American Journal of Evaluation, 24* (4) 423–442.

Sullins, C.D. (2003). Adapting the empowerment model: A mental health drop-in center case example. *American Journal of Evaluation 24* (3) 387–398.

Section

Examples of Three Community Programs Developed by Occupational Therapists

This section describes three community practices developed by occupational therapy doctoral students who incorporated the methods described in Section III. Student projects are an effective approach to starting new community services. Each project evolved from the author's interests and professional expertise and addressed a problem in the surrounding community. Each doctoral student followed the process described in Chapters 7 to 11. Researching for best practices led to development of programs, and financing and marketing activities led to implementation of the programs. Evaluation processes were used to make decisions about each step in program development and implementation, as well as to highlight outcomes of the programs.

In Chapter 12, Fengyi Kuo describes how she combined her expertise in child development and mental health with her passion for social justice and created a program to respond to the needs of children and their families displaced following Hurricane Katrina. Her program and its evaluation have potential to inform future programs for children who are victims of disasters. Chapter 13 describes Ann Chapleau's fortunate contact with an individual working to provide hospice care for people who were homeless. A need was identified for occupational therapy services, which Ann addressed with an innovative program that was valued by clients and other stakeholders. In Chapter 14, Leslie Roundtree describes development of an occupational therapy program for urban high school students who were pregnant and/or parenting. Occupational therapy students were supervised in providing services to these young women using a client-centered approach and occupations important for the high school participants' roles of mother and student.

Each of these programs addresses problems evident in most of our communities. All incorporate client centered, culturally sensitive care while maintaining concern for cost efficacy in meeting community needs through occupational therapy.

Chapter 12

Katrina Kids Program Development and Evaluation

Fengyi Kuo DHS, OTR, CPRP*

IDENTIFYING A COMMUNITY NEED

On Monday, August 29, 2005, Hurricane Katrina made landfall on the U.S. Gulf Coast near New Orleans, Louisiana. The storm brought heavy winds and rain to New Orleans and breached several levees intended to protect the city from the water of Lake Pontchartrain. Consequently, about 80 percent of the city was flooded with water reaching depths near 25 feet in some areas (Pardue, Moe, McInnis, Thibodeaux, Valsaraj, Maciasz, et al., 2005; CDC/US EPA, 2005). The aftermath of Hurricane Katrina caused many thousands of people to be evacuated from Louisiana and Mississippi. In 2006, it was estimated that nearly 5,000 individuals from the Gulf Coast were residing in the state of Indiana due to the impact of Hurricane Katrina

---

*On September 21, 1999, a major earthquake struck Taiwan, causing devastating loss and damage. At the time, I was teaching in an occupational therapy program in the United States and despite the fact that some family friends were impacted by this disaster, I was unable to travel back to my native country to be involved in relief efforts and emergency response. The earthquake took a toll on my family and influenced their quality of life, even years after the earthquake. As a result, I made a personal commitment to be more involved in emergency response, and joined a nonprofit organization as a volunteer. The international charity (Tzu Chi Foundation) organization's mission is to provide compassionate relief during the time of disasters. Volunteering with this organization has provided me great learning opportunities to work closely with community leaders and other stakeholders in their passionate support for the general public during crises.

(Indiana Project Aftermath, 2006). In Indiana, the Red Cross of Greater Indianapolis worked with about 900 families from the Gulf Coast after this natural disaster (Evans & Rockier, November 10, 2005). In the months of September and October 2005, there were about 100 families evacuated from the Gulf Coast to an apartment complex in Indianapolis. It was reported that about 30 of these families remained residents at the apartment complex in August 2006, resulting in approximately 30 to 40 children remaining in the community one year after the storm.

During the aftermath of Hurricane Katrina, I worked with the Red Cross as a volunteer and with a charity organization to distribute emergency relief assistance to Katrina families relocated to central Indiana. In the fall of 2005, I assisted Tzu Chi Foundation in conducting a needs assessment using a questionnaire developed by the organization. The results of the questionnaire indicated that this cohort of Hurricane Katrina evacuees lacked means and financial resources to move to safety and therefore were in the later groups evacuated from the Gulf Coast. Anecdotal conversations indicated that some of the evacuees had moved many times, ranging from two to five different shelters. Their initial stay at the New Orleans convention center was very chaotic and frightening. There was not enough food or clean water. They often could not get enough rest and quality sleep. The evacuees reported that there was constant noise that included babies crying and people screaming. As one evacuee described it, "toward mid-week, some people pulled out their guns and started shooting . . ." (Anonymous, personal communication, September 24, 2005).

It is evident that these evacuees were traumatized. Despite FEMA housing assistance and state funded community outreach counseling, resources to support the evacuees' community engagement, daily living skills, and mental health needs were inadequate. Committed to assisting people who had survived disaster in my community, I developed the Katrina Kids Program to engage young Katrina evacuees in meaningful childhood occupations. The program development and evaluation supported engagement in meaningful and purposeful activities or occupations in order to decrease the impact of trauma on children and their families

LITERATURE REVIEW

The word "trauma" originates from the Greek word meaning "to wound or to pierce." It is a disordered psychological or behavioral state resulting from mental or emotional stress or physical injury. Trauma can occur following war, natural disasters, violence, accidents, or human-caused disasters such as terrorist incidents (Gallimore, 2002). Humans may react to traumatic events with flight-or-fight responses, emotional and psychological symptoms, social dysfunction, and impaired occupational adaptation (Lohman & Royeen, 2002; van Griensven, Chakkraband, Thienkrua, Pengjuntr, Lopes Cardozo & Tantipiwatanaskul, 2006). Severe or prolonged stress following a traumatic experience can impair hippocampal-dependent explicit learning and alter plasticity in the nervous system (Sapolsky, 2003). These neurobiological abnormalities may potentially impact an individual's daily living skills and participation in meaningful occupations (Lohman & Royeen, 2002).

Individuals differ in their capacity to cope with disastrous stress (Friedman, 2006). While some people exposed to traumatic events do not develop psychological distress, others go on to develop severe symptoms. Clinical studies indicate that about 30 percent of trauma survivors develop psychological symptoms or posttraumatic stress disorder (PTSD) (van Griensven et al., 2006). PTSD can turn into a chronic and debilitating condition with varying degrees of impairment. It can disrupt the normal patterns and routines of people's lives. PTSD symptoms can influence a person's occupational balance, including activities of daily living (ADL), instrumental activities of daily living (IADL), education, work, play, leisure, and social participation (AOTA, 2008). Researchers have also identified a delayed variant of psychological symptoms in which individuals exposed to a traumatic event do not exhibit the syndrome until months or even years after the event. Longitudinal research has shown that PTSD can become a chronic psychiatric disorder, can persist for decades, and sometimes may last for a lifetime (Friedman, 2006). Such observations have prompted the recognition that trauma, like pain, is not an external phenomenon that can be completely objectified. The traumatic experience is filtered through cognitive and emotional processes before it can be appraised as an extreme threat. Because of individual differences in this appraisal process, different people exhibit different trauma thresholds.

The devastation caused by Hurricane Katrina, the disaster response, and the preparedness effort are particularly complex (Falk & Baldwin, 2005; Coghlan & Mullins, 2005). The disaster caused enormous physical destruction, environmental deprivation, health concerns, and human suffering (Travis 2005; Pardue et al., 2005; CDC/US EPA, 2005). The sudden displacement of a large population creates a public health emergency (Nieburg, Waldman & Krumm, 2005). Loss of relatives and friends, stress and mental health issues caused by displacement, limited housing, separation from home communities, financial burdens of recovery, and many other factors contribute to difficulty in resuming "normal life" (Voelker, 2005). Those evacuated individuals with resources might be better able to return home or to integrate into a new community, despite the many challenges this process presents. People with limited resources and skills to rebuild their lives face greater challenges. These include the people in constant fluctuation from shelters to hotels to trailer parks or apartment complexes. They are the most vulnerable individuals facing an uncertain future, who will also have the greatest need for governmental and other assistance.

Trauma and disasters change people's lives. Public policy makers, disaster responders, and health care providers should be particularly aware of the most vulnerable populations, whose vulnerabilities are amplified by the stresses and resource shortages that accompany disasters (Nieburg, Waldman & Krumm, 2005). The aftermath of Hurricane Katrina has plainly reinforced the need for addressing health disparities in the United States (Atkins & Moy, 2005; Guidotti, 2006).

Children are frequently the most vulnerable victims of trauma; it is important to understand the impact of trauma on children and to provide intervention to this population. The catastrophic effects of Hurricane Katrina created an unprecedented need for ongoing mental health services to address the impacts of trauma (Voelker, 2005). Occupational therapy practitioners (OTs) can adapt environments to compensate for long-term disabilities caused by natural disasters. OTs can also address mental health issues and help survivors rebuild their lives through participation in valued occupations.

The American Occupational Therapy Association (AOTA) Concept Paper on Disaster Preparedness (Scaffa, Gerardi, Herzberg & McColl, 2006) offers a vision for how OTs can contribute their services during all stages of the disaster process. Many states do not recognize OTs as qualified mental health providers, and OTs are often underutilized in disaster preparedness and response despite the potential need for their services. In addition, a system's infrastructure and limited resources during emergency responses may prevent survivors from receiving services. The Katrina Kids Program demonstrates the role occupational therapy can play in disaster response and recovery by integrating community resources to provide meaningful engagement in purposeful activities to families in need.

In reviewing the literature to implement evidence-based practice, I turned to interventions utilized in trauma studies. Studies support the idea that as traumatized people participate in activities they achieve greater understanding and resolution of their trauma, feel more confident, and are able to trust (Foa, Keane & Friedman, 2000; Gard & Ruzek, 2006). As adults discuss and share how they cope with trauma-related shame, guilt, rage, fear, doubt, and self-condemnation, they prepare themselves to focus on the present rather than the past (Foa, Keane & Friedman, 2000).

A group format provides the ideal therapeutic setting for children to share traumatic material within a safe and cohesive environment. Through engagement in childhood occupations, Katrina youth participants have an opportunity to gain a sense of control over their lives. Group activities may facilitate powerful and therapeutic discussion of psychological, physiological, behavioral, and community responses encountered in the aftermath of a disaster (Norwood, Ursanol & Fullerton, 2000). When a trauma survivor takes direct action to cope with problems, he or she often gains a sense of personal power and control. Active coping means recognizing and accepting the impact of traumatic experiences and then taking concrete action to improve things. Telling one's story (the "trauma narrative") and directly facing the grief, anxiety, and guilt related to trauma enables many survivors to cope with their symptoms, memories, and other aspects of their lives (Foa, Keane & Friedman, 2000).

DEVELOPING THE PROGRAM

Need Assessments

Beginning in September 2005, I volunteered by bringing art and craft activities to hundreds of Katrina evacuees and families housed in Indianapolis. I witnessed the benefits of purposeful activity on social participation and performance adaptation of the Katrina children and their families. After interviewing the families, I decided to conduct a needs assessment as the first stage in planning to expand the activities into an after-school program. I developed an anonymous survey and distributed it at the Katrina Anniversary Gathering in August 2006 to gather recommendations on activities for the program. Stakeholders of the program supported the need for an after-school program for school-aged children with culturally appropriate activities for families and children from New Orleans. One survey participant wrote: "As the educational standards here [in Indianapolis] are much higher than what we are used to in New Orleans, I can tell my daughter struggles a lot with homework; in addition to the trauma we have been going through. I really don't have the ability to help her . . ." (Anonymous, personal communication, August 29, 2006).

Stakeholders recommended the program be offered where they live, either in the clubhouse of their apartment complex or in a local neighborhood library. They recommended it be provided during weekdays, preferably right after school hours when children come home by school bus, sometime between 4 and 6 p.m. Due to a lack of resources to provide transportation home after the program, I decided to offer the program at the apartment complex, where most of the Katrina families with school-aged children could access the services. I then collaborated with the property management firm to arrange a physical space in its clubhouse to offer the program.

Program Preparation

I conducted a telephone survey in preparation for the after-school program. The results indicated that the majority of families who were relocated to Indianapolis during the aftermath of Hurricane Katrina had moved within a year. Some of the families had returned to the Gulf Coast or moved out of the area. Families who relocated to smaller cities in Indiana with major universities have demonstrated higher stability in terms of housing, living arrangements, and employment status (W. Sun, personal communication, November 19, 2006). In November 2006, 29 children, ranging in age from 2 months to 21 years of age, who had moved to Indianapolis in the aftermath of Hurricane Katrina, still lived there. A telephone interview indicated high interest on the part of children, grades 6 to 12, in participating in the after-school program. Due to a lack of transportation and conflicts in work schedules, however, some families were challenged to participate without extra resources or support.

Partial funding for this program was provided by the Indianapolis chapter of Taiwan Buddhist Tzu Chi Foundation and a faculty development grant by the University of Indianapolis, as well as contributions of time and gifts by students and other members of our community. Collaboration among community agencies and organizations, volunteers, and courageous survivors of Hurricane Katrina shows what can be accomplished toward overcoming a natural disaster.

A kick-off party for the program was held in January 2007. During the party, children received winter accessories made by an occupational therapy student, and school supplies donated by Tzu Chi Indianapolis chapter to prepare for the start of a new semester.

Description of the Katrina Kids Program

The aim of the program was to provide meaningful activities to the Katrina children and their families during after-school hours to support their social participation and community engagement. I targeted the program for children in 6th to 12th grades, as a demonstration project to engage young Katrina evacuees in meaningful childhood occupations. Four young Katrina evacuees, whose ages ranged from 12 to 17 years, and their families enrolled in the Katrina Kids Program. I met with the children and their families as a group for 60 to 90 minutes per week for 8 weeks. The Katrina Kids Program included meaningful childhood occupations, such as family interaction, and play and school projects. Culturally relevant activities included creative expression through drawing, and arts and crafts such as making Mardi Gras masks and worry dolls; games; storytelling; and creative writing, such as journaling and writing letters to loved ones. The group sessions usually occurred on Fridays. Occasionally, the group met on Saturdays for outings to explore community resources, including a visit to a cultural exchange event and a dinner at a local restaurant. All participants' families were invited to the community outings to facilitate family interaction. Transportation to the community outings was arranged and provided by the program. In late February 2007, the Katrina Kids Program had its 8-week celebration by visiting The Children's Museum of Indianapolis.

The program started in January 2007, and as a result of its success was extended to include tutoring for children of new immigrants who lived in the neighborhood. I coordinated and trained eight community members to serve as volunteers for tutoring. The tutoring program with math or science activities was offered to all neighborhood kids, ranging from 6 to 15 children, for 2 hours every Thursday and Friday from January to May 2007. Age appropriate activities, such as games and coloring, were provided to young children who did not have school assignments. The clubhouse served as a safe place for neighborhood school-aged children to interact and socialize with each other. At the end of each session, each child received a packet of healthy snacks before going home.

PROGRAM EVALUATION

Mixed method design was used for the program evaluation (Hesse-Biber & Leavy, 2006; Bledsoe & Graham, 2005; Grembowski, 2001; Luo & Dappen, 2005, Greene, Caracelli & Graham, 1989). Both quantitative and qualitative data were collected, primarily focused on the children and families from the Gulf Coast who were participants of the Katrina Kids Program. Three girls and one boy aged 12 to 17 years from two Katrina families participated in the 8-week Katrina Kids Program. Family-Quality of Life Inventory (F-QLI) (Becker, Shaw & Reib, 1997) was administered to both participating families before the beginning of the program. An occupational bingo game was used to gather information on childhood occupations from the child participants. Throughout the program, participants were invited to provide input on the content and activities of the program.

Another tool used for the purpose of program evaluation was the Impact of Event Scale-Revised (IES-R) (Weiss & Marmar, 1997; Weiss, Marmar, Metzler, & Ronfeldt, 1995). The IES-R is a 22-item self-report measure developed to assess current subjective distress for any specific life event. It parallels the DSM-IV criteria for PTSD, with a higher number indicating more severe responses related to PTSD. Results of pre- and post-tests of the IES-R were analyzed using descriptive statistics. The average IES-R post-test was 29 points out of a maximum 88 points, which indicated 9.5 points decrease from the average pre-tests of 38.50 points. Results from three out of four children showed decreased average scores of IES-R on post-tests, ranging from −22 points to +3 points. The difference yielded a positive trend in the children's response to Hurricane Katrina, suggesting that the children may have experienced less negative emotional responses and may have started to have more positive feelings after the 8-week program.

Triangulation was utilized to ensure rigor and trustworthiness of qualitative data, which came from art projects, photographs, field notes, focus groups, and in-depth interviews (Hesse-Biber & Leavy, 2006; Krefting, 1991; Frankfort-Nachmias & Nachmias, 1996; Merriam, 1991). The data provided rich information about the psychological impact of trauma on childhood occupation, the clinical manifestations of such exposure, and effect of the Katrina Kids program. I also utilized member checking and maintained an audit trail to increase trustworthiness of the data (Trochim, 2001; Merriam, 1998). Participants' quotes were presented verbatim to provide rich and thick descriptions in order to enhance transferability of the program evaluation results.

PROGRAM OUTCOMES

As a result of developing and implementing this program, I found that children displaced by a natural disaster experienced loss of friends and meaningful occupations. These losses were partially the result of inadequate resources to stay connected with family and friends living in other distant communities and were compounded by difficulty establishing relationships with peers in their new homes. Cultural differences for program participants who had moved from New Orleans to Indiana also contributed to feelings of loss and alienation in their new homes. These cultural differences included use and meaning of time, valued leisure activities, and community celebrations. The outcomes of this program are described through narratives of participants in this program.

During a home visit to a family, family photos pasted on the wall caught my attention. These included a collection of photos glued on cardboard in which the mother's photo was enlarged and placed on the top, with a family group photo on the middle right. Other family photos were arranged on the wall in cardboard picture frames. I wondered about this grouping of photos. It seemed to me that the cardboard photo frames indicated instability. I then realized that the photos were taken during the first family gathering after Hurricane Katrina. The whole family finally had an opportunity to take reunion photos, after finding out where other members were.

"When were the pictures taken?" I asked.

"Last April [in 2006]." She said.

Eight months after being separated by evacuation from New Orleans, the family was finally able to locate all family members and take pictures of their reunion. I was muted.

Loss and Alienation

When asked about life after moving to Indianapolis, one participant expressed her loss of social community:

"Since mom has not been working, I have to be independent. . . . All of my relatives used to live in the same neighborhood. We just walked around to see each . . . other. We now have family back in Mississippi, my aunt is in South Carolina, and some relatives are in Texas . . . we are all over the place. . . ."

One participant whose house was built near the levee expressed with emotion:

"Some of my family are back there again. But they never thought about coming to get me . . . my aunt went down and took pictures . . . everything was gone."

During a focus group meeting at the end of the program, participants were discussing what one thing they would have taken with them from their home if they had the chance before evacuation. One child responded:

"I want my shoes back. I have that one pair of shoes that I didn't get a chance to pack . . . that was 6:30 Monday morning . . . we were so hurried . . . I just didn't get time to look for my shoes. . . ."

Another participant wished to be able to dance on the streets of New Orleans and talked about how she missed hot summer days. Another participant said:

"I want my whole life back. I want the things to go the way it was, and I wished it all never ever, ever happened. And we would know that the storm was hitting and you know we would've been prepared. If you were prepared you would never have to leave your shoes."

The disaster forced the affected population to relocate to different states across the nation. The long-term evacuation destroyed pre-established community networks and forced a sense of isolation, which is a potential cause of social and occupational deprivation. While talking about rebuilding friendships, one participant stated:

"I don't really hang out with anyone in school . . . I mind my own business. I eat lunch by myself when I go to the cafeteria. I know there are cliques, I just don't get into their circles. I sit by myself and eat my own lunch. I don't really have friends at school . . . kids in my school talk differently, act differently, and do different kind of things . . . I don't really have friends at school."

The same participant continued:

"I don't know . . . I just feel I am different. I really cannot wait to get into college to start all over again. Here many have known each other for a long time, so it is hard to get in as a newcomer. If I would go to college, I would have an equal chance of making friends. Everyone will be in the same position as I am. It will be fair."

The loss of previously established friendships was a common theme in conversations. The relocation due to the impact of Hurricane Katrina created an opportunity to make new friends and rebuild social networks. Challenges remained, however.

"I had many friends who I grew up with at school. I really miss them. There were some friends who I have had since moving here in school, but they have moved back to New Orleans. This kind of friendship is different. It is not the same as the ones you grew up with from childhood. Although we all came from the South, our friendships were new and we didn't have time to grow our relationships. So since they moved back, we haven't really made contact."

The lack of connection can cause emotional distress, which potentially leads to a sense of isolation. When asked whether they have experienced changes in interaction, one participant elaborated:

"Well, in the South, we speak with a different accent . . . They [my classmates] can tell I have an accent. Oh, another is that we say 'country' in the South, but here they say 'suburb'. . . ."

Lack of Resources and a Desire to Return

Families who participated in the program often expressed their lack of resources to connect with their family and friends. This often resulted in lack of activities and meaningful occupations in which they could participate. One participant stated:

"I can't wait for school to start. I am bored at home."

Another participant remarked:

"Most of my friends and family I have not seen since I moved here. This has been hard. There have been some arrangements made and I was hoping to travel south to see my friends. But it never worked out."

One of the program participants needed to check out information on her e-mail account. She indicated a challenge locating a computer with internet access:

"I have so many e-mails in my accounts. I don't even look them up as I really don't have time to access internet while I am at school. There is no way I can do these kinds of things. In school, I have to use the computer to type up my assignments. When I go home, there are no resources like that."

This conversation also alluded to a lack of transportation in the area. While the family lived in the city of New Orleans, family members had easier access to public transportation, which allowed more participation in various community activities.

"I have to take the school bus home. There is no way I can skip that. Last time, I waited an hour for the bus to go to some places."

Participants reported a sense of having lost their original culture, and often mentioned missing family and friends. They wanted to know how things had changed in New Orleans and suggested ways they could see for themselves, rather than rely on secondhand reports of the changes that occurred. One participant asked during an activity:

"Do you think we could take a picture of New Orleans? One day, one weekend . . . or possibly make a trip to New Orleans. . . . All my sisters and my momma have been back, but I haven't. I didn't think that was fair. Everybody else got to see it [New Orleans], but me."

Time

I observed chatting, hugging, and social interaction before the start of each session. If one child didn't show up on time for activities, other children would volunteer to walk over to the child's apartment to find him or her. Once, I walked over with a child to an apartment to find two participants. Upon our arrival, the participants were sitting in their living room watching TV. They welcomed us with open arms. Did they not remember the program would be starting and we would be waiting for them? Did the children lose interest in coming? As Thomas stated in the text *Time, Culture and Identities*, "Time adds a further axis of extension, a further means of defining relations between objects and events . . . time also has to be with us to be capable of inner perception" (Thomas, 1996). Perhaps the participants from New Orleans were living with their temporal phenomena as a part of the culture and daily routines. If I had not walked over to find them or taken initiative to interact with them, they probably would have missed the session. The participants carried their perception of time and culture during the aftermath of Hurricane Katrina. The difference in terms of perception of time became evident when divergence occurred. One participant described her perception of time and routines:

"When I was in New Orleans, my friends and I would just sit on the front porch and talk. We think this is really cool. But here they talk about going to a movie at a certain time, to the mall when . . . we just don't have that type of agenda in the South. This is different."

Meaning of the Program

The Katrina Kids program allowed a group of us to talk, play, laugh, do projects, and process feelings together. Through the project, I witnessed resilience in the children and families from the Gulf Coast. Some families coped. One father stated, "Last year [2005] was very tough. We just had a table, a couple chairs, and a microwave. So we ate frozen food heated up by microwave for Christmas. It was very hard on the kids, too. We have been doing much better this year with my job. We are really starting to enjoy our lives here." The father was able to land a job with his Cajun cooking style. He continued,

"This is like a dream come true . . . with the cooking skills I have . . . if I had stayed in New Orleans, I would have to work 15 more years to get promoted because all other folks know how to cook Southern style food. . . ."

When asked about benefits of the Katrina Kids Program, one participant stated: "I really appreciate all of your help. This is very beneficial to me." Another participant commented on the after-school tutoring:

"I like the program, especially Thursday. It's really good for me because I get my homework done and I get to know a little bit more about people . . ."

One participant spoke of her gratitude:

"I appreciate the people that are doing things for me, taking their time to come help me with my homework and it helps me get through some of my feelings because I talk about my feelings and . . . what I think about like what I'm telling you now."

The children in the program enjoyed making Mardi Gras masks and telling stories of going to City Park and joining parades. One participant hung her mask on her drawer, so she could look at it before she went to bed. One participant used the journal provided through the program to document routines, activities, and emotional responses. Another participant indicated the benefits of making a worry doll during the program: "I did try it and it helps me talk my worries and fears to my worry doll."

Forming a Community Connection: "You are OUR People"

During a community outing to a cultural event, a parent of participants asked me to stop by their apartment after the outing. The mother excitedly requested: "After this event, you have to come by our apartment. You have to take a slice of King Cake before you leave."

King Cake is a special cake served during Mardi Gras and it holds a lot of cultural meaning for the people of New Orleans. After stepping into the kitchen, I saw the cake in a box. Inside the cake was a small plastic baby and the mother explained to me that whoever gets the baby has special privileges and obligations. She cut out the quarter of the King Cake with the baby in it and gave this to me.

"Can I have that? You should keep it for the family." I said.

"Sure you can. Here you go. It is for you with the baby. You are going to be next year's Mardi Gras Queen," she said.

Her little grandson stood by the kitchen looking at us and said:

"Oh! I never had a baby."

"That is for our special Miss Fengyi. You now are OUR people," she said.

I was so touched. I learned people from New Orleans live their culture. That was the moment with the family in their kitchen that I realized I was living in the culture of New Orleans. I kept the slice of King Cake with the baby lying comfortably in the purple, white, and gold colored cake box on my kitchen counter for weeks. I am saving the cake and the baby until next Mardi Gras. Perhaps I might be able to visit New Orleans as a guest with my friends from the Gulf Coast. For them, however, it will be a welcoming home, if they do get to go home.

REFLECTIONS AND RECOMMENDATIONS

Voelker (2005) stated, "Experts warned that Katrina has created an unprecedented need for ongoing mental health services that may not be measured in weeks or months, but years." The results from the evaluation of the Katrina Kids Program supported this statement; children in the program expressed their loss of home, family, friends, and belongings. Although post-test results of IES-R supported the benefits of participating in the program, they also indicated that the children in the program continued to experience high levels of traumatic stress response 15 months after the disaster. Some children in the program became more aware of what they had lost. They realized that the situation was not going away and that they might not return to their "home" anytime soon. They exhibited increased grief reactions. Although a tremendous amount of loss and grief was expressed throughout the program, resilience existed.

As indicated by Mancini and Bonanno (2006), resilience differs from the process of recovery. Resilience in the face of loss or potential trauma is common, and there are multiple and sometimes unexpected pathways to resilience. Future programs for survivors of natural disasters might look into the concept of resilience and investigate how resilience may potentially play a role in trauma recovery.

Organizations and response systems to traumatic events are dynamic systems. Merry (1995), and Priesmeyer and Cole (1995) suggest that disaster responses are nonlinear and disaster organizations often appear to exist at the edge of chaos, which may be a position that allows maximum adaptability. Studies that further support the science of complexity research, such as chaos theory, may be useful in disaster research to develop disaster management techniques and to provide a neuro-occupational perspective on the impact of trauma on human occupation (Abraham & Gilgen, 1995; Priesmeyer & Cole, 1995; Lohman & Royeen, 2002).

The outcomes and processes of the Katrina Kids Program helped me understand the impact of Hurricane Katrina on families, especially on those families who lacked resources to return and rebuild their homes. Issues related to health disparity, occupation deprivation, lack of culturally competent care, and the ineffectiveness of the U.S. healthcare system were evident. Occupational therapy practitioners can be actively involved in emergency preparedness, responses, and recovery and address these issues through the use of occupations. As therapists who support meaningful occupations, it is important for us to support disaster survivors through their grief processes to the reestablishment of structured daily routines, and to facilitate their functional participation in activities that are meaningful to them.

Leading the program provided me an experience of living with the culture of New Orleans. The children in the program taught me how to say "New Orleans" with a Southern accent. They told me stories of Mardi Gras, parades, parishes, City Park, dancing on the street, and what they were missing or had lost, due to Hurricane Katrina. I also learned that it might be valuable to follow up longitudinally with families and children from the Gulf Coast to identify changes in their culture, routines, and life trajectories. Geographic destination of an evacuee may play a role in introducing activities that take place across seasons. "Being able to dance on the street with blues coming out of a balcony" was a frequent request from the children in the program. Adapting to the cold winter season in North America, however, posed an extra challenge for the children and families from the Gulf Coast. Developing new hobbies and interests may be necessary to support balanced leisure activities.

Thomas (1996) describes a past in which time is seen as central to the emergence of identities of people and things. The perception of and use of time is a part of culture. During the course of the project, I experienced the causality and use of time by people from New Orleans. Activities usually started when most participants were gathered. We went by the flow of "here and now," depending upon the current atmosphere. The children and families in the program took the lead in planning for each session. Although I had prepared group protocols for each session, they were used as a working plan for me. It was like dancing the tango. I, the program leader, put the music on and took a step forward, then had an equal share in the role of participation. Once the tone was set and music was on, someone else started to initiate and all took turns to move onto the dance floor. It was extremely fun and dynamic. It was client-centered. Healthcare practitioners working with clients from other cultures without understanding the clients' perception of and use of time as a part of their cultures may expect them to follow a pre-established agenda, which would be a false appreciation of culture and client-centeredness.

It is said that in the city of New Orleans, "Culture is something you live," and "Culture in New Orleans is participatory" (Rutledge, 2006). These statements echo the importance of participation. Upon completion of the Katrina Kids Program, I believe my understanding of people from New Orleans and the impact of trauma from natural disasters are just beginning. David Rutledge (2006) wrote in the book *Do You Know What it Means to Miss New Orleans?* that "The music of New Orleans—like the city itself—is able to move from mood to mood in ways that might surprise people from other cultures. The sense of loss is an inevitable theme . . . but humor, beauty, and the blues all live alongside each other. Even after Katrina, laughter is the best life raft. . . ."

To me, the Katrina Kids Program is a living experience, indicating that many people from New Orleans are still finding their way home. Some of them are perhaps never going to be back home in the South, and some are possibly still looking for a place of comfort where they can keep their culture alive. They may gradually find some place to immerse themselves and in a couple of years call it home. No matter what happens, however, let us not forget about the people from New Orleans, their culture and the touching moments that they share with us. Doing so can inspire all of us to move side by side during the journey of finding home.

REFERENCES

Abraham, F. & Gilgen, A. (1995). *Chaos Theory in Psychology*. Westport, CT: Greenwood.

American Occupational Therapy Association (AOTA) (2008). Occupational therapy practice framework: Domaine and Process (2nd ed.) *The American Journal of Occupational Therapy, 62* (6) 625–683.

Atkins, D. & Moy, E. (2005). Left behind: The legacy of Hurricane Katrina. *British Medical Journal, 331*, 916–918.

Becker, M.A., Shaw, B.R. & Reib, L.M. (1997). *Quality of Life Assessment Manual.* Madison University of Wisconsin–Madison, Quality of Life Assessment Team. [Available: http://www.fmhi.usf.edu/institute/pubs/pdf/qol.pdf]

Bledsoe, K.L. & Graham, J.A. (2005). The use of multiple evaluation approaches in program evaluation. *American Journal of Evaluation, 26* (3), 302–319.

Centers for Disease Control and Prevention/U.S. Environmental Protection Agency. (2005). Environmental health needs & habitability assessment: Joint Task Force. Atlanta, GA: Centers for Disease Control and Prevention and U.S. Environmental Protection Agency. [Available: http://www.bt.cdc.gov/disasters/hurricanes/katrina/envassessment.asp] [Accessed November 10, 2006]

Coghlan, A. & Mullins, J. (2005). The day their luck ran out. *New Scientist, 187* (2156), 8–9.

Evans, T. & Ryckaert, V. (November 10, 2005). Police say abuse followed baby to Indy. *IndyStar Newspaper.* Indianapolis, IN.

Falk, H. & Baldwin, G. (2005). Editorial: Environmental health and Hurricane Katrina. *Environmental Health Perspectives, 114* (1), A12–13.

Foa, E.B., Keane, T.M. & Friedman, M.J. (2000). *Effective Treatments for PTSD: Practice Guidelines from the International Society for Traumatic Stress Studies.* New York: Guilford.

Frankfort-Nachmias, C. & Nachmias, D. (1996). *Research Methods in the Social Sciences.* New York: Worth.

Friedman, M.J. (2006). Posttraumatic stress disorder: An overview. National Center for PTSD. [Available: http://www.ncptsd.va.gov/facts/general/fs_overview.html] [Accessed June 20, 2006]

Gallimore, T. (2002). Unresolved trauma: Fuel for the cycle of violence and terrorism. In Chris E. Stout (Ed.), *The Psychology of Terrorism: Coping with the Continued Threat.* Westport, CT: Praeger.

Gard, B.A. & Ruzek, J.I. (2006). Community mental health response to crisis. *Journal of Clinical Psychology, 62* (8), 1029–1041.

Greene, J.C., Caracelli, V.J. & Graham, W.F. (1989). Toward a conceptual framework for mixed-method evaluation designs. *Educational Evaluation and Policy Analysis, 11* (3), 255–274.

Grembowski, D. (2001). *The Practice of Health Program Evaluation.* Thousand Oaks, CA: Sage.

Guidotti, T.L. (2006). Hurricane Katrina: An American tragedy. *Occupational Medicine (London), 56,* 222–224.

Hesse-Biber, S.N. & Leavy, P. (2006). *The Practice of Qualitative Research.* Thousand Oaks, CA: Sage.

Horowitz, M., Wilner, M. & Alvarez, W. (1979). Impact of Event Scale: A measure of subjective stress. *Psychosomatic Medicine, 41,* 209–218.

Indiana Project Aftermath. (2006). [Available: http://www.projectaftermathindiana.org] [Accessed August 20, 2006]

Lohman, H. & Royeen, C.B. (2002). Posttraumatic stress disorder and traumatic hand injuries: A neuro-occupational view. *The American Journal of Occupational Therapy, 56* (5), 527–537.

Luo, M. & Dappen, L. (2005). Mixed-methods design for an objective-based evaluation of a magnet school assistance project. *Evaluation and Program Planning, 28,* 109–118.

Mancini, A.D. & Bonanno, G.A. (2006). Resilience in the face of potential trauma: Clinical practices and illustrations. *Journal of Clinical Psychology, 62* (8), 971–985.

Merriam, S.B. (1991). *Case study research in education: A qualitative approach.* San Francisco: Jossey-Bass.

Merriam, S.B. (1998). *Qualitative Research and Case Study Applications in Education.* San Francisco: Jossey-Bass.

Merry, U. (1995). *Coping with Uncertainty.* Westport: Praeger.

Nieburg, P., Waldman, R.J. & Krumm, D.M. (2005). Hurricane Katrina: Evacuated populations—lessons from foreign refugee crises. *New England Journal of Medicine, 353,* 1547–1549.

Norwood, A.E., Ursano, R.J. & Fullerton, C.S. (2000). Disaster psychiatry: Principles and practice. *Psychiatric Quarterly, 71* (3), 207–226.

Pardue, J.H., Moe, W.M., McInnis, D., Thibodeaux, L.J., Valsaraj, K.T., Maciasz, E., van Heerden, I., Korevec, N. & Yuan, Q.Z. (2005). Chemical and microbiological parameters in New Orleans floodwater following Hurricane Katrina. *Environmental Science Technology, 39* (22), 8591–8599.

Priesmeyer, H. & Cole, E. (1995). Nonlinear analysis of disaster response data. *Proceedings from Conference, What Disaster Response Management Can Learn from Chaos Theory.* Ed. G. A. Koehler. Sacramento, CA: California Research Bureau, published online, 1996. [Available: http://www.library.ca.gov/CRB/96/05/index.html] [Accessed June 20, 2006]

Rutledge, D. (2006). *Do You Know What It Means to Miss New Orleans?* Seattle, WA: Chin Music Press.

Scaffa, M.E., Gerardi, S., Herzberg, G. & McColl, M.A. (2006). The role of OT in disaster preparedness, response, and recovery. *American Journal of Occupational Therapy, 60,* 642–649.

Sapolsky, R.M. (2003). Stress and plasticity in the limbic system. *Neurochemical Research, 28* (11), 1735–1742.

Thomas, J. (1996). *Time, Culture and Identity: An Interpretive Archaeology.* London: Routledge.

Travis, J. (2005). Hurricane Katrina: Scientists' fears come true as hurricane floods New Orleans. *Science, 309,* 1656–1659.

Trochim, W.M.K. (2001). *The Research Methods Knowledge Base* (2nd ed.) Cincinnati, OH: Atomic Dog.

van Griensven, F., Chakkraband, M.L., Thienkrua, W., Pengjuntr, W., Lopes Cardozo, B., Tantipiwatanaskul, P., et al. (2006). Mental health problems among adults in tsunami-affected areas in Southern Thailand. *Journal of American Medical Association, 296,* 537–548.

Voelker, R. (2005). Katrina's impact on mental health likely to last years. *Journal of American Medical Association, 294,* 1599–1600.

Weiss, D.S. & Marmar, C.R. (1997). The impact of event scale-revised. In J. Wilson & T. Keane (Eds.), *Assessing Psychological Trauma and PTSD.* New York: Guilford.

Weiss, D.S., Marmar, C.R., Metzler, T.J. & Ronfeldt, H.M. (1995). Predicting symptomatic distress in emergency services personnel. *Journal of Consulting and Clinical Psychology, 63* (3), 361–368.

Chapter 13

Occupational Therapy Services for People Who are Homeless and in Hospice Care

Ann Chapleau DHS, MS, OTR

Opportunities to develop an innovative, community-based program can fall right into your lap. If you have identified a community need that you feel passionate about addressing, and you share your ideas or vision with others, sometimes the right people will listen. I was fortunate to have such an experience, which led me to develop a service learning program for occupational therapy students at a residence for terminally ill persons who are homeless. I have worked in the community mental health and addictions field for over 20 years. I have become increasingly concerned by the continued decline in the number of occupational therapy practitioners, and subsequent related services, in outpatient and community-based programs, where I felt our clients had the greatest needs.

In an effort to respond to my growing concern, I recently decided to make a career move to full-time teaching and wanted to be a part of preparing students for varied clinical settings, including nontraditional, nonmedical model sites. I relocated to a large city where I had no contacts in the mental health community, and began teaching mental health and clinical education courses at a small, private university.

IDENTIFYING A COMMUNITY NEED

I worked on expanding our current program's clinical education sites, which were mostly traditional, medical model programs. I wanted students to have opportunities to work collaboratively with community agencies to develop community-based programs. Among other benefits, this would help them develop professional and organizational skills. I was fortunate to work with a fieldwork coordinator who was open to incorporating some of my ideas into the clinical education course for second-year students.

As a new resident in a big city, I began researching community agencies. During my first semester of teaching, I established relationships at a homeless shelter and addiction treatment program. I also contacted a local home health care agency I located through the Yellow Pages. After speaking to the receptionist, my call was transferred to the clinical director. As I introduced myself and began sharing my interest in services that went beyond traditional home health services, she became intrigued.

She described a new facility she had been involved in creating: a residence for homeless persons who were terminally ill. She described the residence as a homelike setting where residents have private rooms and often keep to themselves. Unlike traditional hospice care, persons who have been diagnosed with a terminal illness but have no place to live or no one to care for them are invited to move in immediately, which often leads to lengthy stays. One resident had been at the facility for over two years. Although volunteers provide meals and occasional social activities, the administrator indicated that few organized group activities occurred on a regular basis. She felt the residents could benefit from more meaningful social and occupational engagement. She asked if I would be interested in developing services there.

We spoke on the phone for over 45 minutes. You could say we "clicked." I believe this pivotal moment—this phone call with another person who shared my interests in homelessness prevention and my passion for program development—led to an exciting collaboration. Had I merely politely inquired into home care programs and kept my personal vision out of the conversation, I doubt we would have gotten any further.

Following our conversation, the director referred me to the administrator of the residence. I called her promptly the following day and arranged a meeting and tour. In addition to sharing my ideas with her, I asked her about the needs of the residents, the staff, and management. I wanted to ensure that any services we introduced would be compatible with all relevant stakeholders. We agreed to proceed with a service learning program that would focus initially on a needs assessment of the residents, with a goal of providing recommendations to the staff about activity programming. We both envisioned the first semester as a pilot project that we hoped would lead to an ongoing activity program offered each winter semester.

LITERATURE REVIEW

As I spoke with the clinical director and program administrator, I learned of their concern regarding the limited opportunities for occupational and social engagement of the residents. Our profession is founded on the belief that occupational engagement can lead to improved health and sense of meaning and purposefulness (Yerxa, 1998). In my conversations with the staff, and in reviewing the literature, however, I learned that persons who are receiving hospice care are not routinely referred to occupational therapy because it is viewed as restorative (Frost, 2001; Trump, Zahoransky, & Siebert, 2005). Yet a qualitative study by Lyons et al. (2002), demonstrated that hospice clients who received a broad range of occupation-based activity programming from occupational therapy practitioners in a day treatment program acquired new skills and ways of thinking, and experienced feelings of greater productivity and usefulness.

I encountered another interesting study by Jacques & Hasselkus (2004) that broadened my understanding of the occupational therapy scope of practice in the hospice setting. The authors conducted a qualitative study with hospice recipients and found occupations that challenge occupational therapy's definition of occupation as ordinary, familiar, or daily. The four occupations identified were:

- Continuing life on a daily basis: "Doing the things that matter"
- Letting go: "Getting everything in order and letting go"
- Waiting: "It takes so long to die"
- After death: "A gentle goodbye"

I felt these more inclusive definitions of occupation would be important to share with the students, who would be working to define their role in this nontraditional setting.

DEVELOPING THE PROGRAM

After interviewing stakeholders, reviewing the literature, and using evidence-based practice to guide my planning process, I was able to create a service learning program to meet the identified needs of both students and the local agency. The program also allowed a further opportunity to explore the roles and benefits of occupational therapy in hospice care. Students participated in three weeks of classroom preparation. Lectures provided an overview of community-based and emerging areas of practice, and students learned the consultative model of practice. Additional classroom discussion topics included interdisciplinary collaboration, professional behaviors and ethics, public policy, and advocacy roles.

The First Year

The first year at the residence focused on needs assessment. A group of six students began by participating in the mandatory employee orientation at the hospice facility. Students provided required documentation of current immunizations and CPR training, and completed confidentiality and infection control training. Students then spent three weeks at the hospice meeting with each resident individually, completing the modified Interest Checklist (Kielhofner & Neville, 1983) and developing an occupational profile. Students also interviewed staff to determine program needs. As the final assignment, the students in this first year compiled a manual for the administrator that summarized the results of the needs assessment and included recommendations for programming. They also provided a duplicate manual for me as the course instructor. Student feedback on course evaluations was positive and supported our decision to continue the program the following year.

The Second Year

The following year, our program followed the same general format in providing pre-placement classroom preparation and on-site orientation. Our goal in the second year was to expand the program to include provision of weekly direct services to clients. Students updated the previous needs assessment data with additional interviews of current residents, using a semi-structured format adapted from the Occupational Performance History Interview (OPHI-II; Kielhofner et al., 2004).

Students prepared for their experience by learning to use Goal Attainment Scaling (GAS), a widely used procedure for evaluating the effectiveness of an intervention or program. GAS involves identifying problem areas and goals, using a range of five possible outcomes for each problem, from least to most probable (Kiresuk et al., 1994). Occupational therapy practitioners have used GAS in conducting program evaluation (Ottenbacher & Cusick, 1990) and evaluating client outcomes (Mailloux et al., 2007).

Use of GAS provided structure and guided the students in their planning process. By the third week in the hospice setting, students had worked together to identify three program goals and the possible outcomes of each goal. (See Figure 13-1.) Because the on-site program lasted nine weeks, six additional weeks were available to accomplish all goals. The students had also agreed upon the Model of Human Occupation to guide occupational therapy services in the hospice.

Goal Attainment Scale

Goal Attachment Levels	Activity Resource Book — Goal #1	Participation and Benefit — Goal #2	New Resident Orientation Interest Checklist — Goal #3
Most unfavorable treatment outcome thought likely (−2)	No activity resource manual will be created	Zero resident participation	Nothing is provided for the facility
Less than expected success with treatment (−1)	The activity resource manual will be partially completed	Residents who do participate report no positive benefit from the activity (via survey)	The interest checklist/interview does not meet the needs of the facility and the administration reports negative feedback
Expected level of treatment success (0)	Creation/completion of activity resource manual by 3/24	Half of the residents who participate in the activity report a positive benefit (via survey)	An interest checklist/interview will be provided for the facility to use upon new resident orientation
More than expected success with treatment (+1)	Finish manual ahead of schedule for dissemination with the director and provide an in-service to the volunteers	All of the residents who participate report a positive benefit	The interest checklist/interview will be adopted by the administration
Best anticipated success with treatment (+2)	Volunteers utilize the resource manual before the end of the contracted time (4/7)	All of the residents who are able to participate in the activity do so and report a positive benefit (via survey)	The interest checklist/interview is used by the administration, and volunteers report that this is a helpful resource in establishing rapport with residents

Figure 13-1 The Goal Attainment Scale (GAS) helps occupational therapists evaluate the effectiveness of an intervention or program

Throughout the nine-week process in the hospice setting, each student maintained a reflective journal. The group of students was responsible for submitting a weekly consultation note as well. Students continued to meet weekly in the classroom for ongoing education on topics such as documentation, program marketing, service implementation, evaluation strategies, peer review, and ethical clinical reasoning. Lecture content was timed to roughly match the progression of the community experiences, and class discussions drew examples from community experiences.

I was on site for about half of the community sessions, but was also supervising students in two other community sites. I remained available by cell phone as well, although the students never had a need to contact me. An on-site supervisor was always available—usually the program administrator. All of the staff were aware of the project and were very accommodating. The students generally worked in pairs, taking turns leading and co-leading a weekly group, to avoid overwhelming small groups with too many students. While two students were responsible for each group, the other students were working on the additional projects of preparing a volunteer manual, an in-service, the final paper, and a poster presentation of their experiences. One student commented on her final course evaluation that she appreciated that I was always available but trusted them to act on their own, which she felt allowed for a better learning experience.

OUTCOMES

All three student program goals shown in Figure 13-1 were exceeded. By the time of the volunteer in-service to hospice service providers, which was well-attended, the administrator had already purchased recommended resource materials. In an attempt to match residents with volunteers who had compatible interests, the administrator also had a plan in place to use the modified Interest Checklist as part of the orientation process for both residents and volunteers. The newly hired part-time volunteer coordinator attended the in-service and expressed plans to follow up on the specific activity recommendations.

Student feedback was very positive. I was pleasantly surprised by how interested the students were in the consultation model itself. One student reflected, "This experience has opened my eyes to the need to view the client as the entire [agency], not just the residents." Students also learned the value of flexibility, and how, by simply listening to their clients, they learned how occupation is more than a narrow definition of productive "doing."

"They have stories to tell that I can learn from," wrote one student, "and these stories would have been missed if I didn't make the choice to interact with [clients], even if it wasn't the activity we had planned to do. Sharing what they have is a meaningful occupation for them."

My favorite aspect of the program was the students' final poster presentation. This hospice service learning program was one of six service learning projects occurring throughout the semester. The poster presentation was an opportunity for all the students in the course to learn from each others' group experiences. One of the purposes of this format was to prepare students to publicly disseminate information in a professional forum similar to a state or national conference poster session.

A large room was used to allow all posters to be displayed simultaneously. During the two-hour session, fellow students, faculty and staff, and invited community agency staff from all six sites mingled about, reviewing the posters and participating in the general question-and-answer process. Refreshments were provided, which added to the celebratory atmosphere. Students were professionally dressed and poised throughout the event. Faculty introduced community members to each other, furthering the networking opportunities of the event.

One unexpected positive outcome of the program was the creation of a Level II fieldwork site at the hospice residence. One student, who had become interested in pursuing community practice, requested to complete a rotation there. Working with the academic fieldwork coordinator, I was able to develop the fieldwork manual and complete all necessary agreements. The fieldwork structure is a nontraditional, community-based, nonmedical model, built upon the consultative work completed by the Level I students. I am hopeful that other Level II students will follow, and that by pursuing grant writing opportunities, this facility will be able to fund an occupational therapy practitioner.

REFLECTIONS

There can be as many challenges as rewards to working in community settings. I have experienced many of these challenges in past experiences, when programming did not go as smoothly as it did with the hospice program. I have learned valuable lessons such as to:

1. Establish a solid relationship with administrators and key staff before proceeding, to ensure "buy-in."
2. Provide a guiding structure and literature review that supports the domain of occupational therapy in the setting.
3. Provide a thorough student orientation to prepare students for the unpredictability of program development in community practice.

I believe this program succeeded because of the thorough planning and collaborative process that preceded its implementation. In addition, students were allowed to choose the setting in which they wanted to work; therefore students participating in the hospice program were highly motivated for working with this population and practicing nontraditional roles.

I was flexible and understanding when things did not go perfectly, and because I was comfortable, my students were as well. For example, I prepared students to expect that the weekly groups would never be consistent; therefore, learning to adapt would be crucial. In fact, census was low during most of our time there, and groups were very small. We spent time discussing how to modify planned group activities to accommodate one to three participants, and how to connect with residents who were bedridden and unable to join us in the dining room.

Students had to work through their own grief and loss issues, and we were able to address this in our group meetings, as well as individually through reflective journals. In week two at the site, I had to inform the students that one of our participants had died, shortly after participating in our interview and interest checklist process. In her journal, the student who had worked closely with him was able to reflect on her own personal growth and ongoing goal of coping with loss, which she knew would affect her in any practice setting.

This service learning program is consistent with our profession's vision. One goal of the Centennial Vision is "demonstrating and articulating our value to individuals, organizations, and communities" (American Occupational Therapy Association, 2007). The Centennial Vision calls for expanded collaboration and directs us to strengthen our ability to influence and lead. The ability to both collaborate and lead is crucial to successfully developing community programs that utilize a multidisciplinary approach. Not only did I have to practice both of these skills, but our students did as well. Providing students opportunities to practice a consultative model of service delivery in a nontraditional setting can lead to future community partnerships and more occupational therapy practitioners working in community settings as part of multidisciplinary teams.

The global picture is grand, but the idea is to start small. Find community partners who share your vision, work together to meet the occupational performance needs of your clients, and measure your outcomes. Share your experience with the professional community, which includes, but is not limited to, occupational therapy. As occupational therapy practitioners, our productivity demands are high and our work time is precious, but if you are passionate about your profession's vision, the opportunities are plentiful to be an agent of change in our evolving healthcare environment.

REFERENCES

American Occupational Therapy Association (AOTA) (2007). *Centennial Vision* and executive summary. *American Journal of Occupational Therapy, 61,* 613–614.

Frost, M. (2001). The role of physical, occupational, and speech therapy in hospice: Patient empowerment. *American Journal of Hospice and Palliative Medicine, 18,* 397–402.

Jacques, N.D. & Hasselkus, B.R. (2004). The nature of occupation surrounding dying and death. *Occupational Therapy Journal of Research: Occupation, Participation and Health, 24,* 44–53.

Kielhofner, G., Mallinson, T., Crawford, C., et al. (2004). *Occupational Performance History Interview II (OPHI-II), Version 2.1* Chicago, IL: Model of Human Occupation Clearinghouse.

Kielhofner, G. & Neville, A. (1983). The modified interest checklist. Unpublished manuscript. University of Illinois at Chicago. Available: http://www.moho.uic.edu/images/Modified%20Interest%20Checklist.pdf.

Kiresuk, T., Smith, A., & Cardillo, J.E. (Eds.). (1994). *Goal attainment scaling: Applications, theory, and measurement.* Hillsdale, NJ: Erlbaum.

Lyons, M., Orozovic, N., Davis, J., & Newman, J. (2002). Doing-being-becoming: Occupational experiences of persons with life-threatening illnesses. *American Journal of Occupational Therapy, 56,* 285–295.

Mailloux, Z., May-Benson, T.A., Summers, C.A., Miller, L.J., Brett-Green, B., Burke, J.P., et al. (2007). The issue is: Goal attainment scaling as a measure of meaningful outcomes for children with sensory integration disorders. *American Journal of Occupational Therapy, 61,* 254–259.

Ottenbacher, K.J. & Cusick, A. (1990). Goal attainment scaling as a method of clinical service evaluation. *American Journal of Occupational Therapy, 44,* 519–525.

Trump, S.M., Zahoransky, M., & Siebert, C. (2005). Occupational therapy and hospice. *American Journal of Occupational Therapy, 59,* 671–675.

Yerxa, E.J. (1998). Health and the human spirit for occupation. *American Journal of Occupational Therapy, 52,* 412–418.

Chapter 14

Life Skills Programming for Pregnant and Parenting Adolescent Girls

Leslie Roundtree DHSc, MBA, OTR/L

IDENTIFYING A COMMUNITY NEED

When a friend told me about her new position at an alternative school for pregnant and parenting teenage girls, my first thought was a billboard I saw over 15 years ago with that famous phrase "If only kids came with an instruction manual." As a first time mother in my early thirties, I remember my own feelings of uncertainty and how much of an adjustment to my lifestyle parenting involved. I could not imagine how overwhelming pregnancy and parenting could be for a teenager. Given the complexity of the role of mother and the occupation of caring for others, I immediately began to wonder what types of services were available to these young women. While the education system clearly had identified these girls as a unique population, as evidenced by the alternative school, I was disillusioned to find that the school system directed limited attention to the new skills, responsibilities, and role adjustment associated with being a new parent—especially at such a young age.

Occupational therapy is well established in the school system, where it provides services for children requiring special education due to learning disabilities, developmental issues, and other pathological processes (Brandenburger-Shasby, 2005; Copley & Ziviani, 2004; Maher, Olds, Williams & Lane, 2008; Marr, Mika, Miraglia, Roerig & Sinnott, 2007; Schilling, Washington, Billingsley & Deitz, 2003). Yet it appeared to me that a large population of children—pregnant and parenting teenage girls—are not served within the school system even though their effective participation in life roles, including education, is at risk and susceptible to disruption. Given my interest in health promotion and my practice experience with adolescents in mental health, I began my journey to explore the needs of this unique population and examine the role occupational therapy could play in assisting these young women in adapting to new roles as mothers while successfully completing their education.

LITERATURE REVIEW

The National Center of Health Statistics 2005 data report (Hamilton, Martin & Ventura, 2006), reported an overall decline of 35% since 1991 in the teenage birthrate for women between the ages of 15 and 19. The following year, however, the birthrate for young women ages 15 to 19 increased from 40.5 per 1,000 women in this age group in 2005 to 41.9 (Hamilton, Martin & Ventura, 2007). Ventura (2007) stated, "It is too early to determine if this is a start to a new trend," but given the previous consistent decline this is a worrisome statistic. The Centers for Disease Control and Prevention attributed declining teen birthrates to increased abstinence and improvement in responsible behaviors (condom use) among sexually active teenagers (Ventura, Abma, Mosher & Henshaw, 2006). Yet despite a steady decline, the United States still has the highest teen pregnancy and birth rates among all industrialized countries; rates two to six times higher than most Western European countries (Singh, Darroch, Frost & the Study Team, 2001; Darroch, 2001).

In my research, I uncovered disparities among ethnic minority groups for teenage pregnancy and birthrates. Overall teenage pregnancy has declined among all racial/ethnic groups since 1991, with an overall 42% decline among African-American and a 20% decline among Hispanic teenagers between the ages of 15 and 19 (Hamilton et al., 2006). Nevertheless, according to the Centers for Disease Control and Prevention Department of Adolescent Reproductive Health (2007) Hispanics have an average rate of pregnancy twice that of the national rate, and African-Americans have a rate slightly higher than Hispanics.

Given my interest in my local school district, I explored the state and local rates and found that large urban areas continue to experience disproportionately high teenage birthrates. Each state in my Midwest region has worked diligently to reduce teen birthrates, with current teenage birthrates ranging from 30.3 to 43.3 for every 1,000 women among four states: Illinois, Indiana, Michigan, and Wisconsin (National Campaign to Prevent Teen and Unplanned Pregnancy, 2005). Unfortunately, the birthrates among ethnic minority teenagers in these four states generally exceeded the national average for each ethnic group (National Campaign to Prevent Teen and Unplanned Pregnancy, 2005). Illinois has the tenth highest annual rate for Hispanic teen pregnancies (Illinois Department of Public Health, 2008) and the third-highest rate of all states for teenage pregnancy among African-Americans ages 15 to 19 (Illinois Department of Public Health, 2008). Large urban areas such as Chicago report double-digit teen birthrates of 13.4, while the overall state average is 9.9 (Illinois Department of Public Health, 2004). Consequently, urban school systems serve a significant population of pregnant girls under the age of 18.

I found a growing body of evidence that teenage mothers have lower educational attainment and stagnant economic status growth (Singh et al., 2001; Ehrlich & Vega-Matos, 2000). Cost-analysis reports have demonstrated that teenage mothers are a major drain on the public welfare system, with an estimated $2.3 billion increase in child welfare costs nationwide in 2004, bringing costs to $9.1 billion (Hoffman, 2006). Additionally, researchers have well documented that children of teenage mothers are at risk for preterm birth, low birth weight, developmental delay, and higher rates of infant mortality (Martin et al., 2003; American Academy of Pediatrics, 2001). More recently, researchers have found strong correlations between physical, sexual, and emotional maltreatment among pregnant adolescents (Blinn-Pike, Berger, Dixon, Kuschel & Kaplan, 2002) as well as high levels of depression and loneliness (Hudson, Elek & Campbell-Grossman, 2000).

I discovered that services rarely address the emotional needs of pregnant and parenting teenagers. Most education-based programs continue to focus on family planning, contraceptive education, and abstinence (Amin & Sato, 2004; Hoyt & Broom, 2002). Incentive and mentoring programs have been initiated to help teenage mothers complete their high school education. Many schools and health systems have established case management services to link teenage mothers to community resources for childcare, child development services, health services, and vocational opportunities (Sangalang, Barth, & Painter, 2006). The case management approach provides referrals to community resources (Akinbami, Cheng & Kornfeld, 2001; Sangalang, Barth, & Painter, 2006). The benefits of these resources are evident for the small percentage of teenagers who are able to take advantage of the services while trying to complete their education.

In the state of Illinois, initiatives such as Illinois Early Childhood Prevention Program (Illinois State Board of Education, 2006) offer services to parents of infants and toddlers. These services include parent education workshops, playgroups, monthly home visits, and community referral services.

Unfortunately, only about 23% of teenage mothers take advantage of these services. The majority of that 23% are either not enrolled in school or have not completed their high school education. Only 10.2% of the teenage participants are currently enrolled in high school (Illinois State Board of Education, 2006).

A meta-analysis examining the effectiveness of intervention programs to improve educational attainment among African-American teen mothers revealed that most community based or secondary programs have had minimal impacts, while non-randomized school based programs have had a slightly more significant effect (Baytop, 2006). School based programs using cognitive behavioral approaches were somewhat effective in assisting Mexican-American teen mothers to complete their high school education (Harris & Franklin, 2003). Even with all of the social programs available, I believe society consistently overlooks the disadvantages and risks that early parenting brings to a teenage mother's successful transition to adulthood.

For those teenagers who give birth, schools and healthcare organizations have undertaken limited efforts to provide them with the skills necessary to assume new responsibilities and roles successfully. The primary initiatives in the area of teen pregnancy and parenting continue to focus on deterrent strategies, such as abstinence and the restriction of benefits and support payments to teenage mothers (Singh et al., 2001, Amin & Sato, 2004).

Occupational therapy has taken a very narrow role in assisting mothers, especially teenage ones. Currently, occupational therapy primarily focuses on addressing the limitations of children and educating the parents of special needs children toward facilitating their development (Helitzer, Cunningham-Sabo, VanLeit & Crowe, 2002; McGuire, Crowe, Law & VanLeit, 2004; Olson, & Esdaile, 2000). Overlooked is the large number of teenage mothers with children not identified as requiring special services. A few occupational therapy researchers have completed qualitative studies on perceptions of role competence and role conflict among pregnant and parenting adolescents. While adolescents had positive perceptions about mothering, developmental factors, as well as family and social relationships, shaped their perceptions of their roles and identity as a parent (Levin & Helfrich, 2004; Hermann, 1989; Musick, 1994). I encountered no studies examining the impact of occupational therapy services in assisting teenage mothers to acquire the life skills necessary to assume the new areas of occupation associated with parenting.

The role of mother consists of a variety of responsibilities, including child rearing, home maintenance, meal preparation, health maintenance, and financial management. As described by Esdaile and Olson (2004), mothers as caregivers share co-occupations with their children in a repertoire of social interactive routines between mother and child. These co-occupations, such as playing, feeding/eating, and comforting, require active participation from mother and child. Depending on the age of the teenage mother and her environmental experiences, many of the new expectations require skills that adolescents have not established or that are only emerging on a basic level. (Lindsay, 2000; Milevsky, Schlechter, Netter & Keehn, 2007). Parenting requires the ability to solve problems to address one's own needs as well as the needs of a dependent.

As Larson (2000) points out, mothers use numerous processes and strategies to "orchestrate" the daily parent–child co-occupations. Orchestration refers to processes that require anticipation, forethought, planning, sifting of information, decision-making, balancing, and coordinated responses. Given the complexity of skills needed, it is not surprising that mothers describe motherhood as extremely demanding and overwhelming (Francis-Connolly, 2000). In Francis-Connolly's study (2000), adult women participants had many social advantages: They were married, well educated with college degrees, and most were employed at least part-time. These adult women, however, described themselves as "lacking preparation for the work of mothering" (Francis-Connolly, 2000). It seems unreasonable, therefore, to presume that developmentally immature and socially disadvantaged adolescent mothers can easily assume the responsibilities of motherhood.

Francis-Connolly (2000) reinforces that mothering is a social construct learned through social interactions rather than through biological links. Contextual factors such as economics, social resources, and culture affect how women define and develop roles as mothers. Currently, statistics show that the majority of teenage mothers assume the primary role of child rearing and that practical and informational supports for many are inconsistent (American Academy of Pediatrics, 2001). The literature reports that social support improves pregnancy and parenting outcomes, but there is no consistency in defining social support. Published studies do not take into account variations in need based on the developmental levels of adolescent mothers (Logsdon, Birkimer, Ratterman, Cahill & Cahill, 2002).

Given occupational therapy's focus on person–environment interaction, I felt occupational therapy practitioners were in a unique position to assist pregnant and parenting adolescents. They could help them develop basic decision-making and problem-solving skills related to parenting occupations, and empower them with resources and skills needed to understand and adapt to their new role as mothers. With this perspective, I approached the administration of the alternative school to examine the needs of their population and explore programming possibilities.

PROGRAM PLANNING

This particular alternative school has an enrollment of approximately 200 to 250 students a year. The school provides educational services for 7th through 12th grade. Since this program began, the student population has remained entirely ethnic minority—with approximately 89% of the students being African-American and 11% Hispanic. Ninety-eight percent of the students come from low-income families and approximately 1.7% have limited English skills (Illinois Board of Education, 2005). The young women are between 12 and 19 years old and approximately 11% of the students are in the 7th and 8th grades. In the initial needs discussion, the school's vice principal estimated that at least a quarter of the students have more than one child. As the only alternative school for pregnant and parenting teenage mothers in the metropolitan school system, students come from across the entire city to attend the school. Students receive free public transportation cards through the school for use on the buses and trains throughout the city. Given that the school serves the entire city, I was not surprised to find that the school had only a 49.8% daily attendance rate and that 38% of the students drop out during the course of the school year (Illinois State Board of Education, 2005).

Though pregnant and parenting teenagers can attend any of the public high schools, I found that many of the referrals to the alternative school are by parents who are embarrassed by the pregnancy or by principals who prefer not to have pregnant teenagers in crowded high schools due to liability issues (Miller, personal communication, November 19, 2006). Currently, students cannot graduate from this specialized alternative school but must return to their home school or receive a General Education Diploma certificate. A case manager and special education teacher provide the primary services available for students identified as having special education needs. Currently, approximately one-third of the students at the school are identified as special education students, mainly categorized as learning disabled or as educationally mentally handicapped (Miller, personal communication, November 19, 2006).

The mission of this alternative school for pregnant and parenting girls is to challenge students to achieve academic excellence, while emphasizing prenatal education and parenting skills needed to attain healthy pregnancy outcomes and to train competent young mothers. In addition to academic services and a credit recovery program that helps students make up class failures, the school offered the following support services:

- Homebound services for academic instruction during the period of time when a student is not able to travel to and from school due to delivery or medical reason per physician orders. This service is limited to six weeks.

- Referrals to the Women, Infants and Children (WIC) supplemental food program that provides free food and nutrition information to mothers and their children. This program is a voucher-based access program.
- School social work services to assist teenage girls coping with pregnancy and parenting issues. The school social worker is available in the school one to two days a week. A full-time staff member, known as a student representative, is available five days a week to assist the social worker and students.
- School nurse services are available four days a week to address medical concerns.
- A school psychologist consults with the school once a week and meets with students to address emotional and behavioral issues.

I held individual and group interviews with key and available personnel, including the principal, vice principal, student representative, high school health education teacher, junior high teacher, and school social worker to investigate the perceived needs of the students and the effectiveness of the current support services. The principal identified a health class where curriculum objectives incorporated parenting skills along with general health education most consistent with my program proposal. Through multiple conversations I discovered that even this specialized alternative school offered insufficient education related to the life skills required of a parent. School staff felt a need for targeted services in regard to parenting, general instrumental activities of daily living, and community participation. I discovered that all teachers had the appropriate teaching credentials for their content specialty, but none had specialized training to address parenting issues. The health teacher's background was in health and physical education; when possible, she brought in representatives of community organizations to address child development and other child rearing issues in her class. The specialized service staff, such as the nurse, social worker, and psychologist only provided consultant services to address individually defined problems, and often referred girls to other community services. The student representative had no formal educational background, but had been at the school for over 20 years and was identified as an individual in whom the girls frequently confided.

All of the staff interviewed described the needs of the student population as complex, with personal and environmental issues influencing their success as students and mothers. Many of the students live in chaotic environments. Many care for parents or grandparents who are ill or impaired. Many of the girls come from violent and high crime communities, or from homes where there is a history of violence and substance abuse. A large percentage of the students come from families that lack financial resources for food and other necessities. Additionally, some of the students are homeless; a fair number are wards of the state and live in foster care settings. The school staff reported that family support is very inconsistent and many of the girls have off-and-on relationships with the father of their child or children.

Although school administrators identified only one-third of the teenagers at the school as students with special needs, the staff reported significant behavioral and emotional issues among the students, including fighting, disruptive classroom behavior, depression, suicidal ideation, poor self-esteem, and other emotional disorders. I also discovered a significant number of older girls, 17 to 18 years old, who had accumulated less than ten school credits and still ranked as freshmen. From our discussions, it was apparent to me that many of the girls were struggling academically prior to their pregnancy.

On the average, students remained at the alternative school for a full academic year. Some students, however, have remained as long as two years. The environment is supportive and the staff is very nurturing. All staff interviewed described multiple incidents of spending personal time and resources to assist the students. During my visits, I witnessed the students stopping the staff in the halls with individual requests, and the staff frequently made comments reinforcing the students' presence at school. All of the staff described an open-door policy and reported that the school encourages students to approach anyone if they need assistance. The staff members clearly identified that they knew the school was more supportive and nurturing than traditional high schools, and verbalized concerns about students having the necessary skills to transition back to the general high school population. The school décor emphasized African-American and Hispanic ethnic identity in its artwork and informational boards. In addition, the supportive nature of the environment was evident in the inspirational and self-esteem-boosting materials displayed throughout the classrooms and lunchroom.

When asked directly, key personnel stated the girls needed the most help as new mothers in "parenting skills, survival skills, self-esteem issues, relationship skills, job skills, and use of community resources." The health teacher reported teaching basic child development during the first semester each year. She primarily focused on physical maturation of the child during pregnancy and sexually responsible behaviors.

From the data collected, I hypothesized that the majority of girls were at risk or currently suffering from occupational imbalance, occupational alienation, as well as occupational deprivation. Environmental demands, along with the limited capacity of the pregnant and parenting girls, creates a less than optimal situation or opportunity for engagement in meaningful occupations. According to Wilcock (2006), occupational imbalance occurs when a person's engagement in occupations fails to address individual needs, capacities, or requirements for physical, social, and emotional well-being. Given their current life circumstances, many of these young women are attempting to create a balance between chosen and obligatory occupations—and doing so with limited skills and supports. Occupational alienation results from a lack of satisfaction in one's occupations (Wilcock, 2006). Wilcock (2006) and many other researchers have described how abrupt change, stress, and feelings of meaninglessness can create a sense of detachment. Given that all of the girls have transferred from their home school to a new environment while also undergoing major physiological changes of pregnancy and adjusting to familial and social reactions to their new role of mother, alienation is a strong possibility. Lastly, occupational deprivation occurs when external agency or circumstances keep a person from engaging in occupations of choice (Wilcock, 2006). The complexities of the girls' social environments, as well as economic and institutional restrictions, limit the opportunities for new mothers to fully participate and establish a sense of well-being and competence. I felt, therefore, that an occupation-based life skills program could enhance these young women's ability to engage in their new roles, create a healthy balance, and support future occupational performance.

PROGRAM DESIGN

The primary goal of the life skills program is to enhance the skills of the teenage girls in their new roles as parent and primary provider for their child or children. I defined four overall objectives to guide the program. The objectives are to:

1. Increase the adolescent girl's understanding of activities and responsibilities involved in child rearing and other occupations related to parenting.
2. Assist the girls to establish and improve the performance skills and patterns needed for parenting.
3. Help the girls to develop problem solving skills, decision-making ability, and a sense of self-efficacy in their new roles and responsibilities.
4. Assist the adolescents to locate community resources that support successful engagement in parenting activities.

In collaboration with the school administration, I selected the health class as the best forum for the life skills programming. The State Board of Education learning strategies for physical development and health are broad and allow flexibility of topics. The topics I targeted for the life skills program were consistent with the learning standards and could address three out of the five state learning goals. The targeted state learning goals were (a) State Goal 22: Understand principles of health promotion and prevention of illness and injury; (b) State Goal 23: Understand human body systems and factors that influence growth and development; and (c) State Goal 24: Promote and enhance health and well-being through effective communication and decision-making skills (Illinois State Board of Education, 2006). Given that the life skills program would supplement an existing class, no recruitment of students was required. Because the junior high students did not participate in health class, the teachers and administrators agreed to have them join in during the last session of the day with a small group of high school students.

Although I based my initial program topics on the input from key personnel at the school, I felt it was important for the girls to have an opportunity to express and prioritize their needs before finalizing the design. The students were given the topic list, which included occupations of instrumental activities of daily living, work, leisure, and social participation. I assigned titles to the topics that adolescents could easily understand. During the first week, all students in health classes completed surveys to identify level of interest and to rank their top five topic areas. Many of the girls had difficulty completing the ranking, leading us to aggregate and rank scores for topics in which girls were "very interested." The top five topics were: (1) mother and child bonding; (2) child safety; (3) job hunting skills; (4) goal setting; and (5) helping your child develop through play.

As an educator, I immediately identified this program as an excellent opportunity for community based fieldwork for occupational therapy students. Given my educational program's strong community orientation and its emphasis on the wellness-to-disability continuum, I proposed this life skill program as a Level I fieldwork experience to faculty and administrators of the school. They decided that this was an excellent opportunity for our curriculum's 10-week faculty supervised Level I fieldwork during the second semester of the first year of the occupational therapy curriculum. Two groups of occupational therapy students rotated into this site, each for 5 weeks 1 day a week. A faculty member supervised the occupational therapy students on site. I knew when undertaking this project that it would be impossible for me to assume complete responsibility for its implementation. I recruited a faculty member with pediatric practice experience in the school setting to collaborate on the program's implementation. I served as a consultant to the students, university faculty, and alternative school staff. The fieldwork contract was established and the assistant principal served as the primary site liaison.

Based on topics selected by the girls, each occupational therapy student was responsible for developing at least two group sessions on one of the topics for an assigned class period. Occupational therapy students co-led 30-minute class sessions with each occupational therapy student required to develop a group lesson plan outlining the goals for the session, sequence of specific interactive activities, materials and equipment needed, and questions for process discussion. The occupational therapy faculty supervisor reviewed all group plans prior to implementation. Group plans were required to demonstrate effective use of basic teaching and learning principles, along with use of interactive learning strategies. Students used supplies and equipment from the university to support the group activities. To demonstrate effective teaching–learning strategies, the faculty supervisor led a session entitled "Infant massage—Bonding with baby/child" in each class period. Table 14-1 lists some of the session titles developed by the occupational therapy students.

To enable the occupational therapy students to meet the other objectives of their fieldwork course, the on-site faculty supervisor assigned each occupational therapy student one adolescent girl identified by the social work staff as needing individual attention in one of the defined topic areas. The occupational therapy student collaborated with the adolescent girl to identify one goal to address and set up an intervention plan.

Table 14–1 Session Titles for Life Skills Program.

Child Temperament

Prenatal Yoga

Nutrition

Body Image

Child Safety

Communication Skills

Goal Setting: What do I want to accomplish in the next year/five years?

Time Management: Planning time in my schedule for important occupations

How to conduct myself and answer questions at an interview

How to complete job applications

How do I find good child care?

Helping my child to develop through play

What does my baby's cry mean? What do I do?

OUTCOMES

Occupational therapy students and their faculty supervisor met to discuss the events of each day's service. The health teacher and junior high teacher were encouraged to participate in this session and to give feedback to the students on their leadership and planning abilities. I met with the faculty supervisor each week to review program implementation. Once during the ten weeks, I visited the school to observe the program and seek student and school personnel feedback.

A survey was designed to target the program's goals and topic areas covered. I formatted the questions to discover whether the adolescents felt they had improved their knowledge and performance skills, and whether they could identify relevant community resources to assist them with specific activities in the future. The girls evaluated the life skills program at the end of each 5-week rotation. The faculty instructor instructed the girls not to put their names on their evaluation; a girl in each class volunteered to collect the evaluations and put them in an envelope and return it to the faculty supervisor. The evaluation asked each girl to select statements that best described her learning experience in a specific content session. I listed the titles of each session provided on the evaluation form. Two open-ended questions were asked at the end of the evaluation form regarding what the girls liked "best" and "least" about the sessions. A comment section also was available.

Sixty-five girls participated in the life skills program; twenty-six girls were pregnant and four of those students were pregnant with their second or third child. Thirty-five girls already had a child and three girls had two children. Four girls did not provide any identifying data regarding their pregnancy or parenting status on their evaluations. All class periods had a mixture of ages and educational backgrounds. One class period included the junior high girls. Overall, the girls identified the Life Skills Program as contributing positively to their understanding of the given topics. All five class periods received three of the same topics: infant massage, goal setting, and child safety.

The occupational therapy students led a session on job interviewing skills for all class sessions except the session including the junior high girls. Among the common sessions listed in Table 14-2, the majority of the girls responded that the sessions provided new information about the defined topic. Learning a new approach to a task or activity had the second highest rating. Only four girls (6%) identified five sessions as not providing any new or different information. The girls' negative ratings spread across class sessions, related to different topics, and all occurred during the first five weeks of the program. Seven girls (10%) did not score any of the sessions,

Table 14–2 Adolescent Girls' Ratings of Common Sessions.

	Ratings by Participants				
	Further explained information	Taught a different approach	Provided new information	Made aware of resources	Did not teach me anything new
Infant Massage $n = 64$	26.5%	29.6%	42.1%	32.8%	0%
Goal Setting $n = 55$	21.8%	27.2%	30.9%	29.0%	1%
Child Safety $n = 56$	32.1%	25.0%	33.9%	28.5%	1.7%
Interviewing $n = 30$	36.6%	50%	23.3%	33.3%	3.3%

though they completed the demographic data. Three girls returning to school after the birth of their child only attended and rated one session.

The qualitative data from the open-ended questions on the evaluation regarding what the girls "liked best" was divided between the process and the content of the sessions. Many girls commented on how the occupational therapy students conducted the sessions. They noted that topics were fully explained, a variety of topics were discussed, the activities were fun, and the student leaders were respectful and open-minded. They reported that leaders encouraged all of the girls to talk or get involved. In addition, the girls identified specific content areas that they enjoyed. Many girls identified a specific session during each rotation that they liked, while others made general statements about learning things they did not know or learning something new. The girls made fewer comments about what they liked "least." A couple of girls listed specific sessions on "goals" and "job applications" as their least favorite sessions. There were only two evaluations where the girls reported disliking "everything." Some girls wrote that they did not like the sessions that covered topics they already knew about. At least four evaluations identified a student leader's behavior as the aspect the girls liked least. The comments related to student leaders talking too much or not talking (co-leaders) and not making the topic interesting. A few girls commented on their own behavior or that of their peers as something dissatisfying about the program. Their comments included:

- "Some students weren't as willing to share as others."
- "I came in late so I really didn't hear everything explained."
- "I didn't like that the girls in class weren't willing to participate."

Although the majority of the qualitative data reflected the program's impact on learning and understanding the different roles and responsibilities involved in parenting, numerous comments reflected an individual girl's personal perception of the importance of the information to her life and her ability to use the information. Many girls made comments such as:

- "They taught me things that could help me further on in my life."
- "The sessions were a great example of different things in life you would have to do."
- "Thank you for helping me with some of my future goals."

A couple of girls described the program as confidence building:

- "They taught me things I needed to know and made me more confident."
- "They taught me how it's important to always think about myself positive."

Nevertheless, there were girls who seemed overwhelmed by the information. Their hesitancy was noted in their comments:

- "It was okay but I am not ready for all this."
- "I like least when we were talking about after high school because I am not sure what I want to do but I have some ideas."

Data suggests that the process and the content were relevant to the girls and their new or upcoming roles. By exploring the tasks and occupations associated with their new roles, the girls started imagining themselves in their future life, which assists in shaping identity. As Christiansen (1999) has highlighted, identity, occupations, competence, and meaning are interrelated concepts. Through the things we do we receive validation as being competent. Nevertheless the individual must have his or her own understanding of self and ability within a meaningful context that shapes identity.

REFLECTIONS

The preliminary results of the Life Skills Program for pregnant and parenting teenage girls demonstrate that education focused on the occupational needs and skills of adolescent mothers can help address the girls' capability to deal with risk and overcome barriers to success. Over 90% of the girls believed they learned something from the sessions that targeted responsibilities and skills needed in their new roles as parents and primary providers for their child or children. Anecdotally, both the occupational therapy students and the adolescent girls expressed a broader perception of parenting and the skills needed. Many of the occupational therapy students had children and were young mothers themselves. The girls connected quickly with them, facilitating the acceptance of the Life Skills Program.

Though it was difficult in the school environment to measure actual change in performance, the qualitative data supports the program's influence on student sense of self-efficacy and perception of ability. Perception of individual ability—to affect the environment or assume responsibility—is crucial to occupational therapy. An individual's sense of agency and self-efficacy is critical to creating change and enabling well-being (American Occupational Therapy Association, 2002; Christiansen, 1999; Kielhofner, 2004; Wilcock, 2006; Stone, 2005).

The mixture of ages, educational levels, and current parenting roles—along with the inconsistent attendance of the girls—presented major challenges for program design. These factors also influenced the ability to follow up or build on topics. In addition, emphasizing the relevance of work skills to a successful future seems to need more consideration. While the girls and the school staff both identified work skills as important, the girls did not seem to see these as crucial in their role as parent. Given the social welfare benefits available to young mothers and the uncertainty of parental support, I believe we must explore further the girls' perception of their current need for work.

Addressing the individual needs of select girls during this initial implementation was very difficult due to absenteeism of the identified girls and the schedule conflicts between occupational therapy students and the girls. Nevertheless, it is evident from group sessions, consultation with school personnel, and with the girls themselves that many of the young women have extensive needs that warrant individual attention. I myself wonder how many of these girls with extensive academic limitations and behavioral issues should have been receiving special education services, and why occupational therapy services have not been pursued at the high school level for girls identified as having special needs.

Students' evaluation of the fieldwork indicated the site was initially quite intimidating. Ratings, however, were positive overall. In subsequent fieldwork rotations, the school administration agreed to allow the occupational therapy students to follow select girls to other classes and lunch periods for a more thorough evaluation of their needs and behaviors. During a curriculum revision, faculty also decided that in order to provide greater opportunity to observe and measure impact of the student interventions, occupational therapy students should remain at the at-risk community fieldwork sites for the entire 10 weeks.

The faculty fieldwork supervisor and I have already begun discussions with the school administration regarding the possibility of scheduling education sessions in which the girls would bring their children to school or to the university campus.

As with any community fieldwork experience, the university occupational therapy program supplied the equipment, supplies, and funds for the faculty supervisor. The school administration and I have, however, discussed exploring grants and possibly seeking funding as an instructional intervention under the Response to Intervention of the 2004 Reauthorization of the Individuals with Disabilities Education Improvement Act. The Response to Intervention amendment has a three-tier model, which allows the school to target the entire population of the school, specific at-risk groups, or individuals who are at risk for problems and failure (VanDerHeyden, Witt, & Barnett, 2005). Cahill (2007) has clearly pointed out the role occupational therapy can provide in services to children and adolescents who are at risk for occupational dysfunction. Pregnant and parenting teens are clearly at risk relative to their academic performance and in their new roles as mothers.

After the success of this initial program, I am more convinced than ever that occupational therapy can play a unique role in establishing skills in parenting occupations and in promoting healthy lifestyles and occupations for both adolescents and their children. While national efforts continue to try to reduce the number of teenagers giving birth, occupational therapy can help to curtail the occupational disparities faced by these mothers and their children.

REFERENCES

American Academy of Pediatrics. (2001). Care of adolescent parents and their children. *Pediatrics, 107,* 429–434.

American Occupational Therapy Association. (2002). Occupational therapy practice framework: Domain and process. *American Journal of Occupational Therapy, 56,* 609–639.

Akinbami, L.J., Cheng, T.L. & Kornfeld, D. (2001). A review of Teen-Tot Programs: Comprehensive clinical care for young parents and their children. *Adolescence, 36,* 381–393.

Amin, R., & Sato, T. (2004). Impact of school-based comprehensive program for pregnant teens on their contraceptive use, future contraceptive intention and desire for more children. *Journal of Community Health Nursing, 21,* 39–47.

Baytop, C. (2006). Evaluating the effectiveness of programs to improve educational attainment of unwed African American teen mothers: A meta-analysis. *The Journal of Negro Education, 75,* 458–477.

Blinn-Pike, L., Berger, T., Dixon, D., Kuschel, D., & Kaplan, M. (2002). Is there a causal link between maltreatment and adolescent pregnancy: A literature review. *Perspective on Sexual and Reproductive Health, 34,* 68–75.

Brandenburger-Shasby, S. (2005). School-based practice: Acquiring the knowledge and skills. *The American Journal of Occupational Therapy, 59,* 88–96.

Cahill, S. (September, 2007). A perspective on response to intervention. *School System Special Interest Section Quarterly, 14*(3), 1–4. Retrieved August 23, 2008, from AOTA SIS Newsletter Archives at http://www1.aota.org/sis_qtr/index.asp?QStatus=Y&ID=C

Centers for Disease Control. National Center for Health Statistics. Office of Communication (December 5, 2007) Teen Birth Rate Rises for First Time in 15 Years. Retrieved August 26, 2008 from National Center for Health Statistics News Release at http://www.cdc.gov/nchs/pressroom/07newsreleases/teenbirth.htm

Christiansen, C. (1999). Defining lives: Occupation as identity: An essay on competence, coherence, and the creation of meaning, 1999 Eleanor Clarke Slagle Lecture. *American Journal of Occupational Therapy, 53,* 547–558.

Copley, J. & Ziviani, J. (2004). Barriers to the use of assistive technology for children with multiple disabilities. *Occupational Therapy International, 11,* 229–243.

Darroch, J.E. (2001). Adolescent pregnancy trends and demographics. *Current Women's Health Report,* Oct. 1 (2):102–110.

Ehrlich, G. & Vega-Matos, C. (200). The impact of adolescent pregnancy and parenthood on educational achievement: A blueprint for education policymakers' involvement in prevention efforts, National Association of State Boards of Education.

Esdaile, S.A. & Olson, J.A. (2004). *Mothering occupations: Challenge, agency and participation.* Philadelphia: F.A. Davis.

Francis-Connolly, E. (2000). Towards an understanding of mothering: A comparison of two motherhood stages. *American Journal of Occupational Therapy, 54,* 281–289.

Hamilton, M. & Ventura, S.J. (2006). Births: Preliminary data for 2005. Hyattsville, MD: *National Vital Statistics Report.* Retrieved January 4, 2007, from Centers for Disease Control and Prevention Web site: http://www.cdc.gov/nchs/products/pubs/pubd/hestats/ prelimbirths05/prelimbirths05.htm

Hamilton, B.E., Martin, J.A. & Ventura, S.J. (2007). Births: Preliminary data for 2006. *National Vital Statistics Reports, 56* (7). Retrieved August 20, 2008, from the Centers for Disease Control and Prevention Web site: http://www.cdc.gov/nchs/data/nvsr/nvsr56/nvsr56_07.pdf

Harris, M. & Franklin, C. (2003). Effects of a cognitive-behavioral school-based group intervention with Mexican American pregnant and parenting adolescents. *Social Work Research, 27,* 71–83.

Helitzer, D.L., Cunningham-Sabo, L.D., VanLeit, B. & Crowe, T.K. (2002). Perceived changes in self-image and coping strategies of mothers of children with disabilities. *OTJR: Occupation, Participation and Health, 22,* 25–33.

Hermann, C. (1989). A descriptive study of daily activities and role conflict in single adolescent mothers. *Occupational Therapy in Health Care, 6,* 53–68.

Hoffman, S. (2006). *By the numbers: The public costs of teen childbearing in Illinois* [Electronic version]. Washington, DC: The National Campaign to Prevent Teen Pregnancy.

Hoyt, H. & Broom B. (2002). School-based teen pregnancy prevention programs: A review of the literature. *Journal of School Nursing, 18*, (1), 11–17.

Hudson, D., Elek, S. & Campbell-Grossman, C. (2000). Depression, self-esteem, loneliness, and social support among adolescent mothers participating in the new parent's project. *Adolescence, 34*, 445–478.

Illinois State Board of Education (2005). *Supplemental school report card* [Electronic version]. Springfield, IL: Illinois State Board of Education.

Illinois Department of Public Health. (2008). *African-American Adolescents: Living in a high-risk population.* Springfield IL. Retrieved August 26, 2008, from Illinois Department of Public Health Web site: http://www.idph.state.il.us/public/respect/african_american_fs.htm

Illinois Department of Public Health. (2008). *Hispanic adolescents: Living in a high-risk population.* Springfield IL. Retrieved August 26, 2008, from Illinois Department of Public Health Web site: http://www.idph.state.il.us/public/respect/hispanic_fs.htm

Illinois Department of Public Health (2004). *Illinois teen births by county 2003–2004* (Health Statistics). Springfield, IL: Illinois Department of Public Health. Retrieved January 22, 2007, from Illinois Department of Public Health Web site: http://www.idph.state.il.us/health/teen/teen0304.htm

Illinois State Board of Education. (2006). Illinois Learning Standards Physical Development and Health. Unpublished. Retrieved January 3, 2007, from Illinois State Board of Education Web site: http://www.isbe.state.il.us/ils/pdh/standards.htm

Illinois State Board of Education Data Analysis, & Progress Reporting Division. (2006). *Illinois Early Childhood Prevention Initiative Program FY 2006 Evaluation Report* [Electronic version]. Springfield, IL: Illinois State Board of Education.

Kielhofner, G. (2004). The model of human occupation. In *Conceptual Foundations of Occupational Therapy* (pp. 147–170). Philadelphia, PA: F.A. Davis Company.

Larson, E. (2000). The orchestration of occupation: The dance of mothers. *American Journal of Occupational Therapy, 54*, 269–280.

Levin, M. & Helfrich, C. (2004). Mothering role identity and competence among parenting pregnant homeless adolescents. *Journal of Occupational Science, 11*, 95–104.

Lindsay, J.W. (2000). Teen parents: Straddling the worlds of adolescence and parenthood. *International Journal of Childbirth Education 15*, (2): 5–8.

Logsdon, M., Birkimer, J., Ratterman, A., Cahill, K. & Cahill, N. (2002). Social support in pregnant and parenting adolescents: Research, critique, and recommendations. *Journal of Child and Adolescent Psychiatric Nursing, 15*, 75–83.

Maher, C.A., Olds, T., Williams, M.T. & Lane, A.E. (2008). Self-reported quality of life in adolescents with cerebral palsy. *Physical & Occupational Therapy in Pediatrics, 28* (1), 41–57.

Marr, D., Mika, H., Miraglia, J., Roerig, M. & Sinnott, R. (2007). The effect of sensory stories on targeted behaviors in preschool children with autism. *Physical & Occupational Therapy in Pediatrics, 27* (1), 63–79.

Martin, J., Hamilton, B., Sutton, P., Ventura, S., Menacker, F. & Munson, M. (2003). *Births: Final Data for 2002* (National Vital Statistics Reports) [Electronic version]. Washington, DC: Centers for Disease Control and Prevention.

McGuire, B.K., Crowe, T.K., Law, M. & VanLeit, B. (2004). Mothers of children with disabilities: Occupational concerns and solutions. *OTJR: Occupation, Participation & Health 4* (2), 53–64.

Milevsky, A., Schlechter, M., Netter, S. & Keehn, D. (2007). Maternal and paternal parenting styles in adolescents: Associations with self-esteem, depression and life-satisfaction. *Journal of Child and Family Studies, 16,* 39–47. Retrieved on August 23, 2008 from PsycINFO Database Record.

Musick, J.S. (1994). Grandmothers and grandmothers-to-be: Effects on adolescent mothers and adolescent mothering. *Journal of Infants and Young Children 6* (3), 1–9.

National Campaign to Prevent Teen and Unplanned Pregnancy (2005 data). State Profiles. Washington, DC. Retrieved on August 23, 2008 from National Campaign to Prevent Teen and Unplanned Pregnancy Website http://www.thenationalcampaign.org/state-data/state-profile.aspx

Olson, J. & Esdaile, S. (2000). Mothering young children with disabilities in a challenging urban environment. *American Journal of Occupational Therapy 54* (3), 307–314.

Sangalang, B.B., Barth, R.P. & Painter, J.S. (2006). First-birth outcomes and timing of second births: A statewide case management program for adolescent mothers. *Health & Social Work, 31* (1), 54–63.

Schilling, D.L., Washington, K., Billingsley, F.F. & Deitz, J. (2003). Classroom seating for children with attention deficit hyperactivity disorder: Therapy balls versus chairs. *The American Journal of Occupational Therapy. 57* (5), 534–541.

Singh, S., Darroch, J., Frost, J. & the Study Team. (2001). Socioeconomic disadvantage and adolescent women's sexual and reproductive behavior: The cases of five developed countries. *Family Planning Perspectives, 33,* 251–258 & 289.

Stone, G.V.M. (2005). Personal and environmental influences on occupations. In C. Christiansen, C. Baum, & J. Bass-Haugen (Eds.), *Occupational Therapy Performance, Participation, and Wellbeing* (3rd ed., pp. 93–115). Thorofare, NJ: Slack.

Ventura, S.J., Abma, J.C., Mosher, W.D. & Henshaw, S.K. (2006). Recent trends in teenage pregnancy in the United States, 1990–2002. In *Health E-Stats.* Hyattville, MD: National Center for Health Statistics.

VanDerHeyden, A., Witt, J. & Barnett, D. (2005). The emergence and possible futures of response to intervention. *Journal of Psychoeducational Assessment, 23;* 339–361.

Wilcock, A. (2006). *An Occupational Perspective of Health* (2nd ed.). Thorofare, NJ: Slack.

Index